SARS-COV-2: Molecular Aspect and Detection Approaches

SARS-COV-2: Molecular Aspect and Detection Approaches

Ali Jebali
Seyedeh Elham Sadeghi

ELIVA PRESS

ISBN: 978-99949-8-177-9

Cover Design: Eliva Press
Cover Image: Ingimage
Email: info@elivapress.com
Website: www.elivapress.com

This Eliva Press imprint is published by the registered company Eliva Press Global Ltd. part of Eliva Press S.R.L. Publishing Group

The registered company address is: Pope Hennessy Street Level 2, Hennessy Tower Port Louis, Mauritius
Eliva Press S.R.L. Publishing Group address is: Bulevardul Moscova 21, Chisinau, Moldova, Europe

SARS-COV-2: Molecular aspect and detection approaches

Seyedeh Elham Sadeghi 1 and Ali Jebali 2

1 Department of Nanobiomimetic, Faculty of Advanced Sciences and Technology, Tehran Medical Sciences, Islamic Azad University, Tehran, Iran. Email: elhamsadeghi70@yahoo.com

2 Address: Department of Medical Nanotechnology, Faculty of Advanced Sciences and Technology, Tehran Medical Science, Islamic Azad University, Tehran, Iran. Email: alijebal2011@gmail.com

Table of content

Introduction

In December 2019, a virus A new one called (SARS-COV-2) was reported in Wuhan (China) and shortly after it led to the epidemic of the Covid-19 disease. Unfortunately, almost 2 years after the epidemic, there is still no effective medicine or vaccine with 100% efficiency. Currently, compliance with preventive protocols and timely diagnosis are the main things in controlling the virus. Following the sequencing of the virus genome, diagnosis based on real time PCR was rapidly developed, but this method requires dedicated laboratory facilities and trained personnel. Of course, it should be noted that in this method, special attention should be paid to false negative cases. Of course, the results can depend on the place and time of sampling. For example, the false negative rate is higher in the early stages of infection. An alternative diagnostic platform can be antibody, glycan and lectin based rapid tests. Glycans have not been widely used in rapid tests, but they offer new opportunities and advantages compared to antibody-based systems. Glycans do not require cold chain maintenance compared to proteins and thus are very suitable for emergency situations. Glycans or carbohydrates play important roles in biology, from cell communication to various disease markers. Analysis of data from the 2009 swine flu pandemic showed that viral hemagglutinins have a high ability to bind to $\alpha 2,6'$-sialic acid present in human respiratory tracts. This shows the importance of glycan binding in viral infections. This property of glycans has made it possible to create biosensors for rapid detection of viruses without using nucleic acid detection methods. Corona viruses express the spike glycoprotein homotrimer on their surface, and the binding of sialic acid to the S1 spike protein subunits is crucial for corona virus attachment. Hulswit et al also showed the binding of acetylated sialic acid to human coronavirus and the affinity of this ligand to HKU1-HE strain was also reported. MERS virus spike proteins also bind to surface sialic acids. But any acetylation of sialic acids decreases binding affinity. This evidence shows that the binding of sialic acid is very important in corona virus infection and of course the structure of these glycans can also be important. It has also been found that sulfated glycosaminoglycans (including heparin sulfates) can bind to the spike protein of the coronavirus and prevent the virus from entering host cells. The above examples show that this particular glycan may provide opportunities for the diagnosis and even treatment of covid-19. Of course, it must be said that glycans individually show little affinity for protein targets, but if several glycans are symmetrically placed together, this problem is solved and the affinity increases. This property has also been shown in dendrimers), peptides/proteins, polymers and nanoparticles, and with this principle, strong biosensors can be created for rapid identification of microbial strains without using nucleic acid detection methods.

Corona viruses are from the Coronaviridae family and cause respiratory diseases. One of the newest corona viruses is SARS-COV-2, which causes an infectious disease called the disease COVID-19. The disease of COVID-19 is considered one of the most important viral diseases in the current decade, which has caused a widespread pandemic in the world. Sometimes some corona viruses attack the respiratory system and sometimes they show their symptoms in the stomach or intestines of people. The symptoms of the corona virus in the lungs usually appear in common colds and a type of secretory cold called pneumonia, which is usually a mild cold in most people. In this category, four coronaviruses have been discovered:

HCOV-229E

HCOV-OC43

HCOV-NL63

HCOV-HKU1

These four types of coronavirus regularly cause disease in the human population and cause infection in the respiratory system of people. But there are other types of coronaviruses that have more severe symptoms, such as Sars, MERS and Covid-19. COVID-19 has flu-like symptoms, including fever, cough, shortness of breath, runny nose, and acute respiratory problems. Also, the coronavirus affects other vital organs such as the liver and kidney. Many people who are sick are asymptomatic. The incubation period of the symptoms of this disease was four days. Ground-glass opacity was seen in 56% of cases in chest CT scan. 17.9% of patients with mild symptoms and 2.9% of patients with severe symptoms did not show any problems in their radiology or CT scan.

Studies on SARS-COV-2 began early in the pandemic

SARS-COV-2 is circular in shape and belongs to the family of membrane-bound viruses with positive polarity RNA that infect vertebrates. It contains a genetic material and spike proteins are located on the surface of the virus. SARS-COV-2 has four structural proteins on its surface, which include spike glycoprotein (S), small envelope protein (E), matrix protein (M) and nucleocapsid protein (N). Spike protein (S) is the largest protein on the surface of the virus, which plays an important role in binding to healthy cells and infecting host cells. In fact, the spike protein initiates infection through receptor recognition and membrane attachment and is a key factor in host specificity and interspecies transmission. Spike protein has two regions S1 and S2. S1 contains receptor binding protein domains that bind to cell surface receptors. S2 contains fusion peptides that involve membrane fusion with the host cell. These interact with angiotensin-converting enzyme 2 (ACE2) and can enter human organs such as epithelial cells and damage the vascular system. The first SARS-COV-2 detection method is based on a targeted analyte. There are several biomolecules that are used as targeted analytes such as RNA, DNA, enzymes, and antigens that exist in various bioassays (28).

Diagnosis based on CRISPR

The CRISPR technique is important for optimizing genome editing and therapies, metabolic fluxes, as well as synthetic genetic systems. CRISPR-Cas9 is a molecular device that is used in the fields of genetic and protein engineering. The applications of using this method are genome editing, treatment, diagnosis and gene regulation. CRISPR (Clustered Regularly Interspaced Short Palindromic Repeats) are clustered regularly interspaced short palindromic repeats, which are nucleic acid sequences called CRISPRs. CRISPR technique has wide applications due to its features such as fast, high sensitivity, specificity, accurate, cheap and reliable. This technique is used not only in the diagnosis of COVID-19, but also in the diagnosis of cancer, the identification of single nucleotide polymorphisms (SNPs) and the diagnosis of genetic diseases. Although efficient platforms based on CRISPR-Cas9 have been developed, the discovery of Cas13a (formerly C2c2) and Cas12a (formerly Cpf1), both of which have collateral cleavage activity, has revolutionized the field of nucleic acid detection. As we know that nucleic acids are the main biomarkers for diseases, CRISPR-based diagnostic methods rely primarily on identifying the specific sequence that produces the disease and then cutting that sequence to generate a readable signal. CRISPR diagnostic tests are highly sensitive because most of them use fluorescent probes that are very sensitive. This characteristic of them comes from binding to the target through the Watson-Crick base pairing rule between RNA-DNA or RNA-RNA. The CRISPR technique is fast because it does not require isolation of culture or extraction of genomic DNA. The basis of the diagnosis of this technique is the genome of the virus, that is why this diagnostic method can be used at any stage of infection, especially in the early stages of the incubation period, without the need for confirmatory tests. In the CRISPR technique, using CRISPR-related enzymes and bacterial enzymes, we can identify and cut nucleic acid sequences such as 9Cas, 12Cas and 13Cas. In 12Cas and 13Cas, there are specific enzymes that recognize viral RNA sequences and cut the sequence. To use the CRISPR method, we don't need complicated tools and we can detect COVID-19 using paper strips at the lowest cost and in the shortest time. In this diagnostic method, Csa13a nuclease consists of two different stages: The first step is RT-LAMP (Loop-mediated isothermal amplification), viral RNA is reverse transcribed into cDNA and then amplified using LAMP. The second stage of RNA transcription takes place and is cleaved by CRISPR/Cas13a. In this way, this method can generate a specific sequence in SARS-COV-2. Using the cleavage made in RNA related to SARS-COV-2, we observe fluorescent signals, which shows us that it is COVID-19 positive. The CRISPR method is very sensitive compared to the RT-PCR method, and it is easy, fast, and highly sensitive to detect COVID-19.

Diagnosis based on antibodies

In this diagnostic method, it can be detected even if the person has no symptoms or has already been infected with COVID-19, but in the RT-PCR method, the person may be infected with COVID-19 but without clinical symptoms. In this case, RT-PCR cannot detect the COVID-19 virus because RT-PCR is for detecting the active COVID-19 virus in the body, and only when the virus is actively present in the body can it be detected. Our immune system produces specific antibodies in response to COVID-19. In the early stages of the disease, an antibody called immunoglobulin M (IgM) is produced in the body. In fact, immunoglobulin M is the body's first line of defense, which is produced by B lymphocytes. In the face of N and S proteins, COVID-19 reaches its maximum in the first four weeks and we can measure it for several months. Immunoglobulin M is found mostly in blood and lymph fluid. It is the first antibody that the body makes to fight against a new infection. Antibodies are proteins that are produced by the body's immune system in response to infection and are specific to that particular infection. Also, immunoglobulin G (IgG) is found exclusively in the blood and is the major antibody in secondary immune responses initiated by memory B cells. IgG increases after two weeks after symptoms appear and is a long-term immunity and we can measure it for several months. Immunoglobulin M (IgM) is produced in the blood after the first exposure to the virus, and then immunoglobulin G (IgG) is produced. Immunoglobulin M (IgM) decreases in the blood of infected people after a few weeks, but immunoglobulin G (IgG) is present in the blood after months and even after the person recovers from the disease. In this research, 58 patients were tested in Wuhan, China, and 94% of them tested positive for COVID-19, and both their IgM and IgG antibody tests were positive.

Detection using PCR

Diagnosis of SARS-COV-2 in this broad level of disease requires urgent diagnosis. DNA sequencing methods are often expensive and not cost-effective. But the PCR method (Polymerase chain reaction) is cheaper and takes less time and has high sensitivity. PCR was invented by Kari Mullis in 1983. In 1993, he shared the Nobel Prize in Chemistry with Michael Smith. In PCR types, DNA polymerase enzyme is used, which directs DNA synthesis from deoxynucleotide layers on a single-stranded DNA template. DNA polymerase adds nucleotides to the 3' end of a designed oligonucleotide as it replicates to a longer template DNA. The purpose of PCR is to produce a region of target DNA in order to analyze that gene. In PCR, even if a piece of DNA is present in a small amount, we can produce millions of copies of that piece. In the PCR technique, we use the DNA polymerase enzyme to synthesize DNA on another single-stranded DNA template.

Genome replication is as follows:

In the first step, two strands of DNA are separated and each strand is used as a template to build other strands. In PCR, we need raw materials, including:

1- DNA template: It is a sample that contains the target DNA sequence. At the beginning of the reaction, high temperature is applied to the main double-stranded DNA molecule to separate the two strands.
2- 2- DNA polymerase enzyme: a type of enzyme that synthesizes new DNA strands complementary to the target sequence. Taq DNA polymerase is one of the most common of these enzymes.

In real-time PCR, the transcription is reverse, in this way, before PCR, the RNA of the sample is converted to cDNA by the reverse transcriptase enzyme.

3- Primers: Primers are short pieces of single-stranded DNA complementary to the target sequence. DNA polymerase starts synthesizing the template DNA strand along with these strands.
4- Single units of nucleotides: dNTPs or deoxynucleotide triphosphates such as bases A, T, C and G, which are basically builders of new DNA strands, by being put together, make new DNA strands.
5- Magnesium ion: Doubly positive Mg acts as a factor for the activity of DNA polymerases by causing dNTP mixing during polymerization.

Magnesium ions catalyze the formation of a phosphodiester bond between OH-3 of a primer and the phosphate group of a dNTP. Also, doubly positive Mg facilitates binding between primers and DNA templates by stabilizing negative charges on the phosphate DNA ladder.

6- Buffer: Buffer is a suitable chemical environment for DNA polymerases. The pH of the buffer medium is between 8 and 9.5.

PCR includes the following steps:

1- Initial preparation: Initialization is a reaction that is heated for 2 to 10 minutes at a temperature of 94 to 96 degrees Celsius.

At this stage, DNA polymerase and other reagents are activated and impurities in the mixture are denatured.

2- Denaturation: In this step, the DNA template strand in PCR types is heated to 94°C for 20 to 30 seconds and the hydrogen bonds between the DNA strands are broken and the strands are separated and the DNA is It becomes single-stranded.
3- Binding: The primers are attached to the specific sequence of the DNA template to direct the replication of the DNA polymerase. In the annealing stage, the temperature of the reaction is reduced for 20 to 40 seconds at 50 to 65 degrees Celsius so that the primers are attached to the template single-stranded DNA.

In Annealing, the temperature should not be too high because the primer cannot be connected well, and also if the temperature is low in Annealing, non-specific primers are connected and lead to non-specific amplification. The concentration of the primer in the reaction is much higher than that of the template DNA strand, so primer-template hybridization is much greater than the rebinding of the DNA strands. When the primer binds to the template, DNA polymerase starts incorporating dNTPs onto the template.

4- Elongation: In the extension stage, the reaction is heated to 72 degrees Celsius, which is the optimal temperature for the operation of DNA polymerase. DNA polymerase extends the primers and adds nucleotides to the primer in sequence using the target DNA as a template. DNA polymerase starts incorporating dNTPs in the 5' to 3' direction on the synthetic strand.

The optimal temperature for the elongation of different DNA polymerases is different. For example Taq DNA polymerase normally operates at 72-78°C. The duration of elongation also depends on the length of DNA of the main template, the desired amplicon and the speed of the DNA polymerase enzyme. Normal DNA polymerases polymerize new strands at a production rate of 1 to 1.5 kilobases (1000-1500 nucleotides) per minute.

5- Final elongation: in the final elongation stage (Final Hold), the last stage where the reaction temperature is reduced to 4 to 15 degrees Celsius. This temperature is because until the user removes the samples from the thermocycler, the amplified DNA samples remain intact and do not denature.

For a typical PCR reaction, we need to set the thermocycler in 3 steps of denaturation, binding and elongation in 25-35 repetitions, which takes about 2-4 hours for the whole reaction. If the reaction goes well, we have billions of one or more copies of the target DNA. In order to know that our target DNA fragment has been correctly amplified, we can use gel electrophoresis, which is a quick method to check molecular sizes. The size of the amplified product in PCR types is estimated by using DNA ladder, which indicates the molecular weight containing DNA fragments of known sizes. All these steps are done using a thermal thermocycler or a PCR machine, which replicates DNA with periodic programs and adjusting the temperature. The highest temperature of the thermocycler is 99 degrees Celsius and the lowest temperature is 4 degrees Celsius. The PCR test is performed by sampling the genetic material of the virus called RNA. The PCR test is performed by taking samples from the nose, throat, and saliva with the help of a swab, then the swab is taken to the laboratory to perform PCR. In the laboratory, the desired genetic material is separated from the rest of the sample and placed in the machine. If the test answer is positive, fluorescent light is produced.

Detection of COVID-19 by dogs

Dogs have played an important role in medicine for many years. The smelling ability of dogs that has been used for military personnel. If dogs are trained, they have a great ability to detect the corona virus and are very efficient in detecting possible COVID-19. The positive people of COVID-19 have a specific symptom (specific volatilome) different from non-infected people, which dogs can detect by smelling them. give Evidence of the ability of dogs to detect various types of infections is evident, and the ability of dogs to detect COVID-19 is also being debated. Human sense of smell can also diagnose diseases, especially in the past, this method has been used to diagnose diseases because in ancient times there were no advanced diagnostic tools and humans use this same sense of smell to diagnose diseases. did For example, metabolic disorders in babies and ketoacidosis in diabetics create their own odors. Cancers also have their own odors. Clostridium perfringens (Clostridium perfringens), a skin infection bacterium that is a typical bad smell of gas gangrene. During the Second World War, most doctors used their sense of smell to diagnose infections and diseases because there were not many diagnostic tools available during the war. For example, Pseudomonas aeruginosa infection, which was caused by a wound infection and smelled like a fruit. The nose is used to perceive volatile organic compounds (VOCs). In each of the nostrils, almost inside the skull, there are two covering tissues called epithelium, where the cells of the olfactory nerve are located in the epithelium. Inside the epithelium, in addition to the olfactory sensor cells, there are several other types of cells that are arranged in vertical columns and each one plays a role. The olfactory sensor cells are in the shape of a club with two bundles, the protruding part of which is located in the middle part, and the cell is always in the club part. The bundles of this club are called axons. The lower handle of this club is also called a tooth. Above the epithelium there is a soft tissue, in this soft tissue, axons are connected and form interwoven threads. There is also a gland in this tissue that secretes olfactory mucus. In the lower category, there are villi called flagella, which are always moist with a slimy liquid called olfactory mucus. When we smell something, the molecules of that substance pass over the olfactory epithelium and dissolve in the mucus and reach the fat cells. Smell is a highly developed sense in dogs. A dog's sense of smell is used for both military and civilian purposes. Humans use dog training for their diagnostic purposes. For example, dogs are used in military operations to chase fugitives, find explosives, and find enemy fighters. Also, dogs are used for medical purposes. For example, in America, dogs are trained to diagnose cervical cancer, and they are also trained to diagnose diabetes and epileptic attacks. They have used the sense of smell of dogs to diagnose cancers. One such article tells of a dog repeatedly sniffing a mole on its owner's leg, which later turned into melanoma. It was later confirmed that dogs can detect melanoma. Humans use dog training for their diagnostic purposes. A distinctive response such as barking in dogs when exposed to these markers. For example, when the disease is positive, it is associated with rewarding the dog. In dogs, training is usually associated with rewards. The correct answer is reinforced by giving the dog a ball. In the first step, the dog is introduced to the scent to be tested. In the next steps, by diluting the scent or impregnating it with other substances, they make it more difficult for the dog, and finally the dog is trained to distinguish between positive and negative samples. Basically, the animal's behavior towards a specific smell is associated with a reward. The very good sense of smell of dogs and the ability to condition dogs by humans has caused humans to use dogs for their own purposes, such as finding explosives and missing opioids. The dog's sense of smell is very sensitive and can detect concentrations as low as parts per million (ppm) or billions (ppb).

Volatile organic compounds and diseases

Volatile organic compounds (VOCs) are compounds that have a low molecular weight and evaporate easily at normal temperatures and pressures. Volatile organic compounds (VOCs) are organic chemical compounds that have a high vapor pressure at room temperature. This high vapor pressure is due to the low boiling point of these materials, which causes a significant number of molecules of these materials to turn into gas due to the process of evaporation or sublimation and spread in the surrounding air. For example, formaldehyde has a boiling point of -19 degrees Celsius. Formaldehyde slowly separates from color compounds and disperses in the air. Volatile organic compounds are scattered everywhere. Some volatile organic compounds are natural, such as trees and plants, and some of these compounds are produced by humans, such as perfumes and fragrances. All organs of the human body produce cellular volatile organic compounds (VOC). These volatile organic compounds flow into the blood and are also released into the human environment through breathing, saliva, urine, feces, and skin. When these volatile organic compounds (VOC) are released into the environment is unique to each individual. When these volatile organic compounds are released, their concentration in human breath is ppb to ppt and its concentration in human blood and urine is ppm to ppb, which is constantly being emitted from the human body. The odor specific to each pathogen that dogs recognize consists of a specific pattern. For example, respiratory fluids, aerosols, and volatile organic compounds each have a specific pattern, and also volatile organic compounds are released from the human body. Dogs can detect pathogens by smelling. The organic compounds that are released from the body of people vary, and their concentration is due to genetic differences, environmental settings, diet, drug use, and smoking, which affect the volatile organic compounds that are released from the human body and cause These patterns may be different for each person. So we conclude that the pattern of volatile organic compounds is different under the influence of pathological and physiological processes. Infection in volatile organic compounds (VOC) may be caused by a pollutant or a drug or a drink and food, and finally, volatile organic compounds produced by the human body that have changed their pattern due to an infection or a disease can be a It is a sign to detect that disease by dogs. If we assume that the concentration and nature of volatile organic compounds are different in each infection or disease, then the volatile organic compounds emitted from the human body are under pathological influence. Issues such as neoplasia, infections and metabolic disorders. So the patterns specific to each voc (volatile organic compounds) represent a sign. For example, patterns specific to volatile organic compounds (VOC) may indicate a disease or an infection. such as cancer, diabetes, tuberculosis, irritable bowel syndrome, etc.

Dogs can detect melanoma as well as bladder cancer. Dogs have detected lung cancer from the smell emitted by the exhalation of infected people. In addition, dogs can detect cervical cancer from volatile organic compounds in the cervix, as well as Clostridium difficile in human stool samples. In the same way, dogs can detect diabetes in the exhalation of people with diabetes, keto acidosis 4 and hypoglycemia. So we can conclude that dogs have the strongest sensors to detect pathogens. Now we want to see if dogs can detect the escape of COVID-19 through organic compounds.

Production of volatiles and SARS-COV-2

SARS-COV-2, the causative virus of COVID-19, is one of the single-stranded and enveloped RNA viruses with a diameter of 80-120 nm and is divided into four groups: alpha, beta, gamma and delta. These four coronaviruses HCOV-NL63, HCOV-229E, HCOV-OC43 and HCOV HKU1 are not pathogenic and only cause mild respiratory diseases. But the two corona viruses SARS-COV and MERS-COV are transmitted to humans and cause disease. Corona virus has four proteins in its structure, which are: (Nucleocapsid), E (Envelope), S (Spike) and M (Membrane). COVID-19 uses Angiotensin-converting enzyme-2 (ACE2) as a receptor to infect cells with ACE2 through the second RBD receptor (Receptor-Binding Domain) that is present in Spike protein.

Using saliva to diagnose COVID-19

Corona detection through saliva is also called RT-LAMP. We need a simple, rapid and accessible test to diagnose COVID-19. We found out that the saliva of the mouth is the host of the corona virus. We have a meta-analysis examining the detection of SARS-COV-2 in saliva and examining positive saliva test and oral manifestations. Here we analyze the information extracted from the Meta-Disc software. Since the outbreak of COVID-19, the primary diagnosis of COVID-19 has been through nasopharyngeal swabs. Nasopharyngeal swab is not a suitable diagnostic test because it causes irritation, coughing, sneezing and confusion of the patient. Acute respiratory syndrome of coronavirus in the oral cavity due to the presence of angiotensin-converting enzyme 2 (ACE2), which is the main receptor of COVID-19. that this enzyme is present in the lungs and saliva that the COVID-19 virus can be detected in human saliva up to a month later. We compared the accuracy of detection of COVID-19 by RT-PCR in saliva and SARS-COV-2 by RT-PCR in nasopharyngeal swabs. We have educational ID, country, age, sample size, sample source and number of patients with COVID-19 who were identified through saliva. We also analyzed the statistical analysis of the data including true positives, false positives, false negatives and true negatives of the random effects model in Meta-Disc software. If there is COVID-19 in the saliva, the symptoms are dry mouth, dry and inflamed mouth, enlarged and swollen lymph nodes under the jaw. It was also found that saliva is a biological fluid in which SARS-COV-2 appears. The study of this evidence shows that the detection of SARS-COV-2 through oral saliva has 86% sensitivity and 96% specificity. An example of a diagnostic indicator is COVID-19. These studies show that saliva is the main agent of transmission of COVID-19. Salivary glands that secrete human saliva include proline-rich proteins, mucins MG1, MG2 and gp340. We have 700 microbial species in our saliva, which are oral and systemic microorganisms. The advantages of detecting SARS-COV-2 through oral saliva are that it is easily extracted and also exists in saliva for 20 days or more, and we can detect COVID-19. SARS-COV-2 can be transmitted from person to person directly through coughing and sneezing. There is a large amount of virus in human saliva, especially in the back of the oropharynx. In the studies conducted, it was found that SARS-COV-2 was found in bronchoalveolar lavage fluid (93%), nasal swab (63%), sputum (72%), bronchoscopy brush fibrobiopsy (46%), pharyngeal swab (32%), stool (29%) and blood (1%) are easily detectable and SARS-COV-2 cannot be detected in urine samples.

Binding of protein S to ACE2

Spike is an S-glycoprotein that binds to the integral type I membrane in ACE2; After Spike binds to the type I integral membrane, pH-dependent endocytosis occurs. If pH decreases, the virus loses its cover. Lysosome and endosome become acidic pH, which activates cathepsin B and L enzymes, and S glycoprotein is broken into S1 and S2 subunits. The S1 subunit is responsible for binding to cell surfaces and the S2 subunit is responsible for integrating with the host cell membrane. In order for the virus to enter the cytosol of the host cell, it must be in an acidic environment with a pH of about 3. The virus starts multiplying in the cytoplasm of the host cell using its RNA polymerase and infects the neighboring cells as well. The corona virus creates double-layered vesicles and stops the expression of pattern recognition receptors, which makes the innate immune system unable to recognize them and they continue to multiply inside the vesicle. All of these processes, from the transmission of the virus to the host cell and the pathways of protein expression and the use of cofactors and reagents that pass through the cell membrane, can be identified and recognized in the exhaled breath of people. Also, SARS-COV-2 has a different viral receptor compared to influenza or rhinovirus and produces special volatile organic compounds, and as a result, COVID-19 is distinguished from other viruses. Finally, excessive production of inflammatory cytokines occurs. These cytokines make the immune system work better. Absorption of immune cells to the site of inflammation causes the growth of the site of inflammation and damage to the organs. Inflammatory cytokines secreted by T lymphocytes and macrophages, as well as molecules interleukin 1, interleukin 12, interleukin 18, tumor necrosis factor alpha, interferon gamma, which play an important role in the function of the innate immune system. These inflammatory processes cause a reaction to SARS-COV-2 infection and cause lung damage. Cell structure is destroyed due to oxidative stress and lipid peroxidation and volatile organic compounds, which can increase the destruction. In previous studies, volatile organic compounds were investigated in healthy people and in patients with acute respiratory distress syndrome (ARDS) and it was found that there is a higher amount of n-pentane and a lower amount of isoprene in exhaled air. As a result, these specific volatile organic compounds cause detection. Based on the previous information, we find that dogs can detect COVID-19 by using paraspecific organic compounds that are from body secretions and are a sign of SARS-COV-2. These volatile organic compounds have diagnostic uses. Dogs have been trained in many countries to diagnose Covid-19. In people who are positive for COVID-19, their armpit odor is different from that of people who are negative for COVID-19, and they trained eighteen dogs to detect positive COVID-19 from armpit odor. The trainers taught the dogs that if they consider the smell of an item's armpit to be positive, they should sit in front of it. In a 21-day period, the trainers trained the dogs and the detection success rate was from 83% to 100%. This has been a sign of their success. Cases of dogs were declared positive for COVID-19 before their RT-PCR results were positive. In addition, to detect COVID-19, we need a method that is less time consuming and less expensive than the PCR method. This high detection rate led the researchers to the conclusion that dogs can be trained to detect COVID-19 in a short time. In these countries, including the United States, eight dogs are being trained to detect COVID-19 through the smell of samples infected with the corona virus. In Chile, dogs are being trained to detect COVID-19 through the sweat samples of infected and healthy people. to identify These dogs can be used as biological detectors of COVID-19. These tests made us realize that dogs can identify positive people with COVID-19 by being trained to smell the secretions that come out of the human body. It should be kept in mind that there must be positive and negative examples for training dogs. To train dogs, we must be careful that the volatile organic compounds that cause the dog's response or the dog's detection are not related to a specific place or time. For example, specific organic compounds that are associated with a specific location. We need a test that is fast, efficient, non-invasive, and also cost-effective to detect COVID-19 for the reopening of schools, airline travelers, and religious congregations, which we believe is a viable solution using dogs.

A review of previous studies

Quing et al. described the distinct role of sialoside and its receptor protein in coronavirus infection. They found that virus particles attach to cells and this is done with sialic acids. Viruses first bind to sialic acids and then bind to protein receptors. Overall, these findings suggest a role for sialic acids in virus attachment and protein-directed cell-cell fusion and enhancement of corona infection.

Hulswit et al demonstrated that human coronaviruses OC43 and HKU1 bind to 9-O-acetylated sialic acids through a conserved site located in the spike protein. Both viruses use receptors based on sialic acid as a key component. These data enable the investigation of the evolution and pathobiology of OC43 and HKU1 and open new avenues for preventive and therapeutic interventions.

Kwon et al claimed that sulfated polysaccharides effectively inhibited coronaviruses in vitro. They showed that heparin has a good affinity to bind to the spike protein of the coronavirus. They proved that this molecule can be used for treatment and follow-up.

Jeyaram et al showed in molecular dynamics simulation studies on influenza A H5N1 virus that sialic acid and sialic acid fluorine bind well to the corona virus and have a good ability to bind for diagnostic and therapeutic purposes.

Sun et al explained the role of sialic acids on the cell surface to cause corona virus infection. It is thought that sialic acids on the host cell surface can also act as co-receptors for SARS-CoV-2 cell entry. Computer modeling and molecular modeling predictions showed that sialic acid has a potential role in virus binding and entry. In vitro and ex vivo studies on sialic acids also confirmed these findings.

Tabari et al used computer simulations to combat COVID-19. Computer simulations and related data play an important role in drug discovery and development. In this context, antiviral drugs, herbal chemicals, anti-inflammatory agents were used using molecular modeling, molecular dynamics (MD) and the results show that the promising effects of such compounds are used in experimental and clinical trials. Takes. Chloroquine, chloroquine-OH and amifenovir as virus entry inhibitors, Remdesivir, Ribavirin, Lopinavir, Ritonavir and Darunavir as viral replication inhibitors, and Sirolimus are examples that after comprehensive evaluation of available data in molecular simulation It has been tested on patients.

In a study by Alfassam et al., sialic acid-conjugated gold nanoparticles (SA-Au NPs) were used to detect SARS-CoV-2, the influenza B virus, in patients. SA-Au nanoparticles had an average particle size of 30 nm and negative zeta potential of 30 mV. These nanoparticles had the ability to change color after coming into contact with contaminated samples. This research shows that this nanostructure is a quick and simple diagnostic tool that can be used for rapid virus detection.

In their review article, Mehdi and colleagues point out the importance of using nanoparticles in the diagnosis of corona virus and treatment of covid-19. Nanoparticle-based strategies to fight this virus have great potential. It can also be very effective in diagnosis, treatment and vaccination, which requires more research.

In their study, Abo-Zeid and colleagues succeeded in showing the binding of iron nanoparticles to the binding domain of the spike protein in the coronavirus. This study showed that both Fe_2O_3 and Fe_3O_4 nanoparticles effectively interact with SARS-CoV-2 S1-RBD. Fe_3O_4 forms a more stable complex with S1-RBD. These interactions are associated with structural changes of viral proteins and as a result viral inactivation.

SARS-COV-2 detection methods

COVID-19 has remained at the center of attention since the pandemic. March 2020 Due to the rapid and uncontrollable spread of COVID-19 worldwide, diagnostic tests are the first line of defense against human-to-human transmission of this infectious disease, with reverse transcription polymerase chain reaction (RT-qPCR) being the gold standard. To demonstrate high sensitivity and specificity in the diagnosis of SARS-COV-2. However, alternative tests are being developed and capitalized on due to global demand for the facilities, reagents, and healthcare staff required for rapid population-based testing. Also, the rapid evolution of the viral genome and the emergence of new types necessitates the updating of existing methods. The goal of scientists is to improve the tests in order to be cost-effective, simple, fast and at the same time accurate and efficient, as well as user-friendly testing. Current diagnostic methods are either molecular based that detect the abundance of nucleic acids, such as RT-qPCR and reverse transcription loop-mediated isothermal amplification (RT-LAMP), or immunologically based that detect the presence of antigen or antibody in Patient samples, such as Enzyme-linked immunosorbent assay (ELISA), lateral flow assay (LFA), chemiluminescence immunoassay (CLIA) and neutralization assay. In addition to these strategies, sensor-based or CRISPR applications are promising tools for SARS-COV-2 detection. This review summarizes the latest updates in SARS-COV-2 detection methods with their limitations. Researchers, epidemiologists, and physicians are identifying a faster, more reliable, and more sensitive method for diagnosing SARS-COV-2. Severe acute respiratory syndrome coronavirus 2 (SARS-COV-2) is a positive single-stranded RNA virus that caused the novel coronavirus disease 2019 (COVID-19) pandemic. According to the World Health Organization (WHO), about 604 million people were infected, with more than 6 million deaths worldwide by August 2022.

(WHO, 2022; COVID-19 Map, 2022) The disease is highly contagious and can It can spread rapidly to the respiratory tract through close contact with infected people through talking, coughing, and sneezing. Most patients suffer from symptoms ranging from fever, cough and fatigue to mild to moderate pneumonia, while a few require hospitalization and mechanical ventilators. High-risk groups – the elderly over 65, the obese, patients with chronic diseases, or immunocompromised patients – may develop serious complications, leading to septic shock, multi-organ failure, and death. On the other hand, some patients do not have any symptoms. But it can still spread the disease to others. Studies have yet to report any significant differences in viral loads between asymptomatic, presymptomatic and symptomatic patients, as reviewed. However, other studies reported a positive association between high viral loads and symptom severity. (Walsh et al., 2020) This virus has significantly surpassed the spread of Sars and MERS, both in terms of the number of infected people and in terms of the geographical spread of the epidemic. (Hu et al.,2021) Moreover, this crisis, which emerged in late 2019, continues to affect today and poses a tremendous threat to public health and socioeconomics on a global scale. The unpredictable effects of genetic changes (mutations) on functional proteins can worsen this situation in the near future by changing the nature of the virus in terms of its transmissibility and infectivity. Also, asymptomatic people are estimated to be 75% more likely to spread the disease than symptomatic cases, potentially driving the spread of the virus out of control. In order to prevent this epidemic, extensive and widespread testing is crucial to limit the uncontrolled spread of the disease. Quantitative reverse transcription polymerase chain reaction (RT-qPCR) was declared the gold standard by WHO. However, this method requires expensive and precise instrumentation in laboratory environments operated only by experienced personnel, which is very challenging to achieve the number of tests per day compared to the available resources. Alternative methods for simple and rapid on-site testing are needed to cover larger populations in resource-limited areas or to address global demand for diagnostic reagents and equipment. Therefore, researchers are continuing studies to develop rapid, cost-effective and practical solutions for the detection of new SARS-COV-2. In this review, we summarize recent advances in sampling and diagnostic methods to identify a faster, more reliable, and more sensitive method for diagnosing SARS-COV-2 infections. Based on recently published findings, the genome organization and emerging variants of SARS-COV-2 and clinical applications such as sample selection, serological and molecular techniques for virus identification are comprehensively reviewed.

Genome organization of SARS-COV-2 and emerging variants

Known coronaviruses originate from animals. Some of them can co-exist with humans (human coronaviruses) as local infections with low pathogenicity (HCOV-HKU1), HCOV-OC43, HCOV-NL63, (HCOV-229E), while others such as corona Severe acute respiratory syndrome virus (SARS-COV), SARS-COV-2 virus and Middle East respiratory syndrome virus (MERS-COV) cause severe diseases in humans with mortality rates of 9.10%, 1.2% and 3.34% respectively. % have evolved. SARS-COV-2, together with SARS-COV and MERS-COV, belongs to the genus Betacoronavirus, a family of Coronaviridae with high genetic diversity. (Wang et al., 2020) With a size of 9.29 kb, the SARS-COV-2 genome consists of open reading frames (ORFs) that encode ORF1ab polyproteins at the 5' end; and the regions encoding nucleocapsid (N), membrane (M), coat (E) and spike (S) structural proteins at the 3' end. The S protein consists of the S1 subunit, which contains a receptor-binding domain (RBD) that binds to the angiotensin-converting enzyme 2 (ACE2) receptor on host epithelial cells; and the S2 subunit, which mediates viral fusion and entry into host cells. Also, SARS-COV-2 genome has 16 non-structural proteins (nsp) in which nsp12 encodes RNA-dependent RNA polymerase (RdRp). This enzyme catalyzes the synthesis of RNA from an RNA template and is thus responsible for viral replication. Like many viruses, SARS-COV-2 underwent genetic mutations or changes that emerged from the original "L" strain from Wuhan, China in late December 2019. The nucleotide mutation rate of SARS-COV-2 genome is estimated as 4.67710-6 substitutions per site per year. (Wang et al., 2022), which reduces the effectiveness of detection techniques. The emergence of new types and the high mutation rate of the viral genome require updating the existing diagnostic tests. Since the start of the pandemic, WHO has tracked and documented genetic lineages that provide clear evidence of risk to global public health through increased transmissibility, infectivity, or reduced effectiveness of diagnostic tools, treatments, and vaccines. WHO describes lineages with these characteristics as varieties of concern (voc). On the other hand, other SARS-COV-2 strains with genetic mutations that have globally equivocal evidence of increased transmissibility, disease severity, and immunogenicity are referred to as strains of interest (vol). Currently, there are no vols in circulation until August 2022. shows global SARS-COV-2 strain labels and their scientific nomenclature, mutations, first date of appearance, and documented origin according to WHO and Centers for Disease Control and Prevention (CDC), with the predominant VOC Omicron . Other species previously identified as voc are now downgraded to species under monitoring (VBM). Whole genome sequencing of Omicron species revealed more than 30 amino acid mutations in the S gene, the majority of which are in the RBD. As described by (Venkatakrishnan et al., 2021), the Omicron genome acquired a unique three amino acid insertion (ins214EPE) not previously observed in any of the SARS-COV-2 lineages. It is assumed that such an insertion in the genome can be possible by a pattern change mechanism. In this model, the exchange of genomic material between the genome of the host (human) and the genome of the virus (SARS-COV-2) and another viral genome (such as human coronavirus 229E (HCOV-229E)) is possible. With this variant, a higher risk of reinfection was reported compared to the others due to its increased ability to evade host immunity. SARS-COV-2 can be detected in various samples such as swabs (nasopharynx, oropharynx and anus), saliva and sputum. The virus can also be found in other body fluids such as blood, urine, and feces. This is due to the high expression of ACE2 receptors in the cells of blood vessels, kidneys and intestines. (Salamanna et al., 2020) In addition, the expression of transmembrane protease, serine 2 (TMPRSS2), an enzyme that cleaves the S protein of SARS-COV-2 and significantly accelerates virus entry, in the respiratory system , the digestive system, kidneys and bladder are expressed. (Al-Kuraishy et al., 2021) Sample collection is a very important method for screening for COVID-19 infection in the population. Screenings are conducted in hospitals and distributed testing centers to allow for widespread testing. Such tests are essential to limit the spread of disease, especially in asymptomatic individuals, and to protect healthy individuals from infection, which is why sample collection must be accurate, rapid, and accessible to large populations.

Nasopharyngeal swabs (NP) are long Q-tips inserted into one nostril through the nasal passage to collect samples for the diagnosis of infectious diseases. This technique is the most used with a sensitivity that reaches 98%. (Wang et al., 2020; CDC, 2022) This is considered the gold standard for collecting SARS-CoV-2 samples safely and conveniently because there is no direct contact between the doctor and the sample. In this procedure, patients are asked to tilt their head upwards to insert the swab horizontally through the nasopharyngeal canal. The swab is then held for a few seconds to absorb enough samples. After that, the swab is gently removed while rotating and the tip is placed inside a tube. The applicator is then discarded by cutting it to separate the tip. However, this technique is painful and leads to pain and discomfort for patients. (Butler-Laporte et al., 2021) In addition, it requires technical expertise and healthcare providers must be protected with personal protective equipment (PPE) for sample preparation as close contact with the patient is required.

In addition to NP swabs, oropharyngeal (OP) swabs target the oral cavity and reach the posterior wall of the oropharynx to collect the sample. The tip is rotated several times, then removed and placed in a tube. The applicator is then discarded to remove the cotton piece. This procedure is generally easier and less painful for patients. However, it is less sensitive than NP swabs (Wang et al., 2020; Khiabani and Amirzade-Iranaq, 2021) and the clinician should avoid contact of the swab with the tongue, palate, or uvula during sample collection. Therefore, using a tongue depressor may help guide the swab along the passageway. (Coden et al., 2020) As with NP swabs, receiving OP swabs requires close contact with patients, so the use of PPE is critical.

Few studies have used rectal swabs for the diagnosis of covid-19. (Abdullah et al., 2021; Li et al., 2021) However, its use as an independent test is not recommended. Also, these swabs cause patient discomfort, and researchers are unsure whether these swabs are necessary for population testing. (Dutch Welle, 2021)

Further research has proven that SARS-CoV-2 RNA is present in feces (Liet al., 2021; Lin et al., 2020b; Ling et al., 2020; Xiao et al., 2020) because the virus can It will pass. It targets the digestive system and ACE2 receptors, which are abundant in the epithelial cells of the lungs and intestines. The virus can remain in the patient's stool samples for weeks after recovery. Hence, these samples can determine whether a person has already been infected with the virus.

Unlike NP and OP swabs, saliva sampling is non-invasive and patients do not experience discomfort. Samples can be collected by patients themselves by pouring their saliva into a container and handing it to a healthcare provider. Saliva testing is simple, inexpensive, and readily available because it allows rapid testing of a pooled sample. (Tan et al., 2021; Wei et al., 2021b) Even though there is no direct contact with patients, saliva samples carry increased risks of infection when used by health care providers. Saliva samples were found to have more RNA copies per milliliter than NP swabs, with slightly higher sensitivity in detecting SARS-CoV-2.

NP swabs or saliva samples still contain SARS-COV-2 RNA in asymptomatic patients. (Aoki et al., 2021) However, the sensitivity of this method can be affected by the collection process and sample homogeneity - pure saliva or mixed with mucus or sputum. One study showed a sensitivity and specificity of 73.1 and 97.6%, respectively, when saliva samples were collected from patients at screening centers and used the gold standard as a reference. (Senok et al., 2020) while another study reported a sensitivity of 91%, indicating that saliva is a reliable sample for the diagnosis of COVID-19. Since this technique is non-invasive, it provides an easier opportunity to test children.

SARS-COV-2 RNA can be detected in other types of samples, including sputum, collected from the lower respiratory tract of patients experiencing severe cough. It had a much higher sensitivity of 91.6%, a better indicator of longer-lasting viral load. (Khiabani and Amirzade-Iranaq, 2021; Ravi et al., 2020; Yu et al., 2020) In addition, blood samples contain viral RNA at lower loads, (Li et al., 2021; Ling et al., 2020; Xiao et al., 2020) while most reports did not detect it in urine samples, as reviewed by Walsh et al. (Walsh et al., 2020) On the other hand, feces have been reported to have a higher detection rate (53.42%) because ACE2 and TMPRSS2 are abundantly expressed in the gastrointestinal tract. (Salamanna et al., 2020; Al Kuraishy et al., 2021; Xiao et al., 2020) These additional samples can be used for confirmatory experiments or to further study the virus infection pathway, rather than an independent sample for diagnosis. The types of samples mentioned above are variable in terms of diagnostic accuracy. Sample collection or handling, the amount of viral load in the sample, the severity or time since the onset of infection are all factors that affect the accuracy of the diagnosis. (Coden et al., 2020; Abdullah et al., 2021; Ling et al., 2020; Senok et al., 2020) Some researchers noticed changes when testing different samples from the same patient. (Li et al., 2021; Xiao et al., 2020; Senok et al., 2020). SARS-COV-2 is located in the lungs (lower respiratory tract), not the upper respiratory tract, when the disease begins. Hence, samples taken from this device may show negative results. (Li et al., 2021) Samples with higher viral loads and sensitivity, such as NP swabs and sputum, should be considered to avoid exposing healthy individuals to infection due to false negative results. (Khiabani and Amirzade Iranaq, 2021)

Common methods in SARS-CoV-2 detection and their characteristics such as sensitivity, limit of detection (LOD), detection time, advantages and limitations are summarized. These methods are divided into five methods: 1- based on ddPCR, RT-qPCR and RT-LAMP 2- based on sequence, and 3) serological methods (CLIA, LFA, ELISA and neutralization method), 4- CRISPR technology, and 5) based on biological sensor. The critical points of each method are explained in the following sections.

Molecular based methods

Since its advent, quantitative reverse transcription polymerase chain reaction (RT-qPCR) was the first validated standard technique for the detection of SARS-CoV-2. RT-qPCR is a molecular diagnostic technique that detects the presence of nucleic acids by targeting and amplifying specific genes, resulting in millions of copies of a small number of nucleic acids that can be monitored in real-time. Primers are one of the key components in this reaction because they bind to the target gene on the DNA strand. They must be well designed with high specificity to avoid non-specific binding and unwanted structures such as primer dimers, which can lead to false positive results. DNA probes or fluorescent dyes such as SYBR green show the presence of the desired gene. SYBR green is a dye that binds to all double-stranded DNA (dsDNA) and produces a fluorescent signal. On the other hand, probes contain a fluorescent reporter that binds to the 50′ end and a quencher that binds to the 30′ end of a specific target in DNA. When the enzyme DNA polymerase cleaves the probe, the released reporter emits a fluorescent signal that the device detects. Prior to the reaction, viral RNA is isolated from the collected sample using commercially available RNA extraction kits. This is very important because proper sample handling and avoidance of contaminants will ensure accurate results. Then, complementary DNA (cDNA) is synthesized using master mix containing reverse transcriptase enzyme. The mixture is then incubated in a thermal cycler to initiate the reaction. Afterwards, the cDNA, primers, distilled water, and DNA probe or Cybergreen are pipetted into a 96-well plate and placed in an RT-qPCR machine with appropriate thermal cycler settings. A negative control should be used to confirm the absence of contaminants and to avoid the interpretation of false positive results, which is essential for the diagnosis of COVID-19 patients. A positive control should also be used to avoid the interpretation of false positive results. In general, reproduction is achieved through three basic steps:

1-Denaturation: where the temperature is increased to separate dsDNA.

2-Connection (annealing): In this step, the temperature is reduced and the primers are allowed to connect to their desired sequences.

3-Extension: In this step, the temperature increases again and allows DNA polymerase to extend the primer by adding nucleotides to the new DNA strand.

This procedure is repeated about 40 times and after each cycle new copies of DNA are created. Each time the probes are released, a fluorescent signal is produced or Cybergreen binds to newly synthesized dsDNA. Hence, the intensity of the fluorescent signal increases with increasing DNA copies after each cycle. Ct or cycle threshold values indicate the number of cycles required for the intensity of the fluorescent signal to exceed a predefined threshold. Samples with a higher viral load will have a lower Ct value. Conversely, higher Ct values indicate low amounts of RNA copies in a given sample. RT-qPCR is the gold standard for the diagnosis of COVID-19 because it is rapid, accurate, and specific in detecting and amplifying SARS-COV-2 RNA. (Bustin and Nolan, 2020). Highly sensitive primers and probes have been developed in different countries to target genes such as E, N and RdRp. (D'Cruz et al., 2020; Tombuloglu et al., 2022). Many researchers use similar approaches when identifying SARS-COV-2, and many are trying to overcome some limitations. Kudo et al. (2020), for example, Kudo et al. used a multiplex RT-qPCR with primer probe sets targeting N1 and N2 genes, as recommended by the US CDC. is, to identify SARS-CoV-2 from saliva and NP59 swabs of sick and healthy individuals. They included human RNase P (RP) as an internal control in the reaction. They found that the technique was highly efficient and sensitive as it could detect low viral RNA copies, and concluded that it saved time, reagents and cost. (Kudo et al., 2020) Also, some others used primers targeting the E gene and the RP gene as an internal control along with non-nucleus water for the non-template control (NTC), while 466 healthy samples and They tested the infected. They obtained Ct values ranging from 13.38 to 34.65 for positive samples, indicating the accuracy of the method and the need to use internal controls to validate the results. RT-qPCR technology is undoubtedly specific and sensitive in the diagnosis of COVID-19, hence the gold standard. However, this equipment is expensive and should be used by experienced and trained users, as possible contamination can affect the sensitive RNA extracted from the samples. Also, considerable time is required to obtain results, which adds to the limitations when underdeveloped countries with limited resources require widespread testing for COVID 19. It has been reported that RT-qPCR was either unable to detect SARS-CoV-2 in samples with low viral load or resulted in Ct values greater than 35–40. As a result, these patients can be tested negative, putting them and their families at risk of infection. In addition, global demand for kits, instruments, reagents, trained personnel and even sample collection tools leads to shortages in some regions, necessitating the need for an alternative testing method. To avoid false positives, multiple assays were useful even in case of viral mutations. (Kudo et al., 2020) reported reduced detection sensitivity when testing different RT-qPCR assays on Omicron-type positive samples, particularly those targeting the mutated region. Therefore, SARS-CoV-2 mutations should be screened closely and RT-qPCR assays should be optimized and updated accordingly. (Chen et al., 2022; Sharma et al., 2022). Creating a standard curve using internal controls such as RP and negative control ensures the accuracy of the results.

Droplet digital PCR (ddPCR)

This technique was previously developed to reduce the limitation (Hindson et al., 2011) of false negative results reported in RT-qPCR because it can detect small traces of DNA. This device divides the samples into thousands of drops of water-oil emulsion, each of which has a PCR reaction. This is done by placing the cartridge containing the PCR mixture into a droplet generator. Then the drops are pipetted into a 96-well plate and placed in a thermal cycler. Injection of the spacer liquid then separates each droplet to be identified as positive or negative based on fluorescent signals. Unlike expressing results in relative Ct values like RT-qPCR, ddPCR provides the absolute number of gene copies in a sample using Poisson statistics. Furthermore, studies agreed that ddPCR is more sensitive and specific in detecting SARS-CoV-2 in samples with low RNA abundance. (Behera et al., 2021; Falzone et al., 2020) For example, a study that compared the accuracy between RT-qPCR and ddPCR when targeting the ORF1ab and N genes showed that 26 samples tested in RT -qPCR were negative, they were positive in ddPCR.

(Suo et al., 2020) Similarly, Yu et al. targeted ORF1ab and N genes in different samples showed that ddPCR performed better in virus detection in samples with low viral load. (Yu et al., 2020) However, ddPCR requires sophisticated, expensive instrumentation and takes longer than RT-qPCR to provide results. Another molecular method for the detection of COVID-19, which has attracted the attention of many scientists due to its simplicity and high specificity, is reverse transcription loop-mediated isothermal amplification (RT-LAMP). This simple, rapid and highly specific technique detects viral diseases by targeting and amplifying six regions in DNA, using 4-6 primers. They include forward and backward internal primers and forward and reverse external primers, designated as FIP, BIP, F3, and B3, respectively, in addition to forward and reverse loop primers (LF, LB). (Alhamid and Tombuloglu, 2022) Compared to RT qPCR, RT-LAMP is a single-tube reaction that requires a single enzyme, coupled with reverse transcription, and is performed at a constant temperature of 60-65 °C. Therefore, it does not require a thermal cycler, providing a less expensive alternative to point-of-care testing while maintaining sensitivity and specificity. (Notomi et al., 2015). In this method, an RNA sample is separated from the sample and converted to cDNA by reverse transcriptase enzyme through BIP binding. The RT-LAMP reaction is started in the same tube containing the DNA polymerase, primers, and other substrates, and then placed in a 60-65°C incubator for 15 minutes to 1 hour until the results are obtained. During the reaction, primer B3 binds to its complementary region and initiates complementary polymerization, displacing the cDNA strand synthesized by BIP. FIP binds to the released cDNA strand and similarly initiates displacement and polymerization. he does. Then, the F3 primer outside the FIP binds to its complementary region, and polymerization starts from there, eventually forming dumbbell structures that harbor complementary sequences at both ends. DNA synthesis then begins in the loop regions, releasing millions of target stem-loop DNA sequence structures of various lengths and inverted repeats. The RT-LAMP technique is currently being used to test for COVID-19. Several reports proved its high specificity against SARS-CoV-2. (Aoki et al., 2021; Thi et al., 2020; de Oliveira Coelho et al., 2021; Bokelmann et al., 2021; Lu et al., 2020). Results from RT-LAMP should be confirmed by comparing them with the gold standard RT-qPCR. (Thi et al., 2020) Due to the large number of primers, the possibility of formation of primer dimers increases, which leads to false positive results. This is why primers must be well designed to specifically target the genes of interest. A study compared 19 primer assay sets and found that primer sets targeting the N gene had the fastest amplification and higher sensitivity in the detection of SARS-CoV-2. (Dong et al., 2021) However, in another study, other primer sets targeting the N gene had a Ct of about 35 and showed lower sensitivity than the E gene primers. (Thi et al., 2020) As with other methods, the use of negative and positive controls ensures accurate results. This technique offers simple detection methods including colorimetry, fluorescence, turbidity, and gel electrophoresis, which are reviewed in the following sections.

One of the simplest detection methods in the RT-LAMP reaction is colorimetry, which depends on the pH change as an indicator. This method is the most convenient because the results are visible to the naked eye through the color change. Phenol red, neutral red and cresol red are among the most common indicators that are added to the reaction. Colorimetric kits are commercially available and ready to use to give results in a short period of time. If there is a positive sample, the pH will decrease and the color will change depending on the dye used. This color change can be measured by measuring the absorbance at wavelengths of 434 nm and 560 nm using spectrophotometry. Many reports have used this method for its simplicity and the fact that expensive equipment such as real-time fluorescence is not required, making this diagnostic method cheap, accessible and suitable for point-of-care testing (POCT). For example, one study used a commercially available kit to target the N and ORF1a genes using RT

LAMP colorimetry, which ultimately resulted in a color change from red to yellow in positive samples. They hypothesized that samples with Ct < 30 showed a strong color change at 30 min, while samples with Ct > 30 did not change color or did so after 35 min when tested in RT-qPCR. Additionally, they determined their results by measuring optical density (DOD) at 434 and 560 nm wavelengths. (Thi et al., 2020) Another study to assess specificity identified RdRp and E genes with various respiratory viruses, including other coronaviruses, and no false positive results were obtained; That is, no cross-reaction was observed. They concluded that their results had a sensitivity of 200 RNA copies with a Ct <30. The results were also quantified using spectrophotometry. (Aoki et al., 2021) Others used the cresol red marker and observed a clear color change in samples with higher viral copies in less than 40 min, while samples with lower RNA copies showed very weak color change or They needed a longer reaction time to achieve results.

This detection technique showed promising results, but still has limitations. When the reaction temperature exceeded 65 °C, a color change in NTC was observed, indicating that high temperatures increase the chance of formation of primer dimer structures. Poor results were obtained in RT-LAMP colorimetry with low viral RNA loads and Ct>30. The sensitivity of the RT-LAMP colorimetric method depends on the days when the symptoms of the disease appear. Five days is reported to be the best time for this technique to provide the most accurate results, while sensitivity decreases if more than seven days have passed since the onset of symptoms. (de Oliveira Coelho et al., 2021) Some samples with Ct > 30 require more than 30 minutes of reaction time to cause a color change. However, increasing the reaction time to more than 30 min may result in amplifications that are not specific and lead to false positive results. (Aoki et al., 2021) Both of the previously mentioned studies observed inconclusive results when there was a lower viral load in the sample – i.e., an orange color was produced – testing positive in RT qPCR, indicating another limitation. (Aoki et al., 2021; de Oliveira Coelho et al., 2021). The use of internal controls to evaluate the performance of primers to avoid false negative results, such as the use of human RNA from the MCF7 cancer cell line as a negative control. (Aoki et al., 2021) In addition, the addition of samples directly to the LAMP colorimetric reaction should be avoided, as they cause false positive results due to changes in pH.

RT-LAMP fluorescence

The fluorescence detection method measures the intensity of the fluorescent signal or amplification by adding a dye such as SYBR green to the samples and placing them in a fluorescent detector or qPCR instrument. Bockelman et al detected both the N and Orf1a genes using RT-LAMP fluorescence in less than 30 min and used Cybergreen dye to induce color change. (Bokelmann et al., 2021) Another study used a fluorescence assay to detect the N gene from 157 NP swabs, where positive samples produced a sigmoid fluorescent signal and showed a sensitivity of 87%. Also, the specificity of RT-LAMP against SARS-CoV-2 was tested with other common respiratory viruses through fluorescence detection. After 50 min, only SARSCoV-2 samples resulted in amplification of the fluorescent signal, while others did not, concluding that the technique is highly selective for this virus.

This method measures the deposition of magnesium pyrophosphate, which is a byproduct of DNA synthesis, using a real-time LAMP turbidity meter. Therefore, magnesium pyrophosphate is an indicator. (Notomi et al., 2015) The sensitivity of this detection method has been reported to be 20-200 copies in 60 minutes when using primer sets targeting Orf1ab and S genes. The change in turbidity can be observed with the naked eye or measured by a real-time turbidimeter by measuring the DOD at 650 nm, where positive samples have turbidity values < 0.1. (Yan et al., 2020)

Agarose (2% W/V) prepared with ethidium bromide dye is widely used. Samples are usually loaded into the gel, and positive samples appear as DNA bands that can be visualized under a transilluminator (illuminator). This method detects the presence of DNA after the RT-LAMP reaction (Notomi, 2000) and confirms the results obtained from other detection techniques (Thi et al., 2020). For example, de Oliveira Coelho et al. (2021) confirmed their RT-LAMP colorimetric results by loading their samples onto gels. Samples that showed a color change from pink to yellow appeared as banded patterns under UV light. The detection accuracy increases if there are more RNA copies in the sample. (Aoki et al., 2021)

Sequence-based methods

The scientists used whole-genome sequencing methods to determine the origin of SARS-CoV-2, distinguish it from other respiratory pathogens, and identify emerging variants that occurred in multiple countries through multiple sequence alignments. Whole genome sequencing is the first method used to detect and identify mutations in emerging VOCs including Omicron. Currently, more than 12 million complete genome sequences of SARS-CoV-2 variants have been submitted to the Global Initiative for Sharing All Influenza Data (GISAID) EpiCov database by researchers worldwide. Next-generation sequencing refers to newer techniques that are cheaper and less time-consuming than standard Sanger sequencing, as individual DNA fragments are sequenced in parallel using small volumes on small panels. The principles of next-generation sequencing have already been reviewed. (Slatko et al., 2018; Dorado et al., 2019) Many researchers have sequenced RNA obtained from SARS-COV-2 patient samples of COVID-19 (after being re-transcribed into DNA) to further study the virus and develop treatment options or vaccines. For example, Ren et al. identified S, N and RdRp genes in five patient samples using next generation sequencing. They distinguished the virus from other respiratory viruses and confirmed their results with the gold standard technique. They found 79% and 51.8% sequence homology with SARS-CoV and MERS-CoV, respectively, and concluded that the virus is a CoV of bat origin after performing multi-gene analysis. (Ren et al., 2020) Another study identified S gene mutations associated with increased transmission by whole-genome sequencing of the virus. These studies demonstrated the robustness of SARS-CoV-2 genome sequencing for surveillance. However, these techniques are time-consuming and expensive because they require special equipment and are therefore not suitable for point-of-care testing (POCT). Furthermore, due to the large number of cycles and data generated in the software, they can provide inaccurate results when detecting long sequences.

Today, antibody tests are widely used to determine whether a patient has previously been infected with or is immune to COVID-19, as it detects the presence of antibodies or antigens in the serum, namely immunoglobulin G (IgG) and immunoglobulin M (IgM). Immunoglobulin G is the most abundant neutralizing antibody and remains in the blood continuously from two weeks to four months after the onset of illness, while IgM is produced earlier and declines more rapidly. On the other hand, IgA can be detected in the early stages of infection (within five days) and persists longer. (Tantuoyir and Rezaei, 2021; Padoan et al., 2020) However, these tests do not determine whether patients are currently infected, as the results will be either false negative when their immune system has not yet produced antibodies. , or will be false positive in patients who have already recovered from COVID-19 but whose blood is still producing antibodies. These methods have a high specificity for SARS-CoV-2, ranging from 96.93 to 99.91% compared to the gold standard. It is variable. Regarding sensitivity, a proposal for combining IgG and IgM rather than detecting one without the other seems to be the best choice. (Vengesai et al., 2020) Most assays target the most abundant viral proteins S and N to test for antibodies, (Tantuoyir and Rezaei, 2021) and other assays are coated with antibodies to target a specific antigen, the latter of which detects COVID-19. Serological assays are numerous, but those reported for anti-SARS-CoV-2 antibodies or viral antigen detection include the following.

Enzyme-linked immunosorbent assay

ELISA method is the most popular serological method to detect the presence of antigens, antibodies and proteins in clinical samples. It is widely used in laboratories to test antibodies against SARS-CoV-2 in exposed or recent immunity. Some commercially available assays include SARS-COV-2 recombinant S and N proteins targeting IgG and anti-SARS-CoV-2 IgG using S1. The sensitivity and specificity of the first test were reported as 85.7% and 98.5%, respectively, while the sensitivity and specificity of the second test were reported as 80% and 100%. Samples were tested three weeks after disease onset, symptomatic patients produced higher levels of IgG than asymptomatic samples, and IgG titers in both groups decreased significantly after 140 days (Iruretagoyena et al., 2021) in This test involves adding the patient's whole blood or serum to a plate containing the viral protein. If antibodies are present, they bind to the antigens and form complexes, and those unbound antibodies are washed away. Then, the enzyme labeled with horseradish peroxidase antibodies is added and binds to the antigen-antibody complex. After that, the plates are washed again. Finally, the addition of a substrate leads to an enzymatic reaction that produces color. This color change indicates a positive sample and can be detected by a screen reader. (Behera et al., 2021) others developed a reproducible protocol for SARS-COV-2 protein S-coated ELISA assay that can detect and measure IgG antibodies. (Vernet et al., 2021) Similarly, to detect viral antigens in patient samples, ELISA plates are coated with antibodies specific for SARS-CoV-2 viral proteins. If a person is infected with COVID-19, the viral antigens bind to the coated antibodies and form antigen-antibody complexes. Enzyme-labeled secondary antibodies and a substrate are then added to bind to the antigen-antibody complex and produce a color. This test is known as sandwich ELISA.

Lateral flow assay

In addition to ELISA, the lateral flow method (LFA) detects SARS-CoV-2 antigens. This is a qualitative test that uses blood, swabs, or saliva from patients to detect antibodies or viral antigens. This detection method is based on the principle of immunochromatography. A liquid sample is loaded onto a sample pad and flows into a conjugate pad that contains lyophilized (frozen and dried) reagents, including non-specifically labeled antibodies that bind to antigens. Then, antigen-antibody complexes flow through a nitrocellulose membrane into the test line and are captured by antigen-specific antibodies. After binding, a visible color is produced. A control test line is also available to capture non-specific labeled antibodies to ensure that the sample has successfully passed through the test pads. (Abduljalil, 2020) This assay is simple and does not require laboratory equipment and is therefore A quick point-of-care test, or POCT, is convenient because it takes 15 to 30 minutes to get results. A study developed a small LFA strip to detect the N-antigen of SARS-COV-2 in patient samples using specific antibodies immobilized on the surface of the strip. Their assay had a low detection limit of 0.65 ng/mL. (Grant et al., 2020) Also, LFAs are used to detect antibodies in clinical samples and to identify both SARS-COV-2 anti-IgG and SARS-COV-2 anti-IgM in two separate test lines. that bind to a SARS-COV-2 conjugated surface antigen, in addition to the control test line break, was developed. In this study, they used whole blood samples loaded onto a sample pad and then transferred to a conjugation pad that contained gold-conjugated SARS-CoV-2 antigen. After that, the formed antigen-antibody complexes were moved through a nitrocellulose membrane containing anti-human antibodies. When antigen-antibody complexes bind to anti-human antibodies, a color is produced that indicates the presence of IgG or IgM. They reported 88.66% sensitivity and 90.63% specificity.

Chemiluminescence immunoassays (CLIA)

Chemoluminescence immunoassay (CLIA) relies on the release of energy in the form of light in a chemical-immunological reaction. A luminescent molecule is an indicator that emits a visible light signal due to the transfer of electrons to the ground state after a reaction. There are direct detection methods that use luminophore molecules as markers, or indirect methods that use enzymatic markers with their associated substrates. These markers produce fluorescence signals in relative light units that quantify antibodies in a sample (Cinquanta et al., 2017). These assays detect IgG and IgM against SARS-CoV-2 from patients' serum. Samples are incubated in plates containing magnetic beads with N antigens to form antigen-antibody complexes. Then, enzyme-labeled anti-human antibodies are added and the plates are incubated for binding. Those unbound antibodies are washed away. Finally, a luminescent substrate is added to produce light that indicates the number of antibodies present in the samples by a photomultiplier. This assay has been reported to have a sensitivity of 84.81% and a sensitivity of 91.25%, requiring only 23 minutes to obtain results (Lin et al., 2020a). Others used a similar approach and reported high sensitivity and specificity (Lu et al., 2020). Another study detected IgG and IgM antibodies in COVID-19 patients using multiplex electrochemiluminescence immunoassays coated with SARS-CoV-2 S antigen, in addition to other coronaviruses, to assess the specificity of this technique. A stronger antibody response was observed against SARS-CoV-2 compared to other coronaviruses, indicating high specificity.

Neutralization assays

These assays test the ability of antibodies to block the RBD of the SARS-CoV-2 S protein from interacting with ACE2 receptors on host cells, thereby inhibiting viral infection and replication. In this test, diluted patient serum or plasma is mixed with fully functional SARS-CoV-2, incubated and added to Vero E6 cell cultures. After incubation, the plates are stained, left for a few minutes and then washed with ethanol. Antibodies bound to the viral RBD were determined by reducing plaque formation in cell cultures by 50% and 90% compared to control (Abe et al., 2020). This technique is time-consuming as it requires days to obtain results and must be performed in a level 3 biosafety cabinet due to the high risk of infection. Nevertheless, this technique is very important in vaccine development. (Carter et al., 2020) developed an assay similar to ELISA, but using the binding domain of protein S as antigen and human ACE2 together with the enzyme and its substrate as indicators. ACE2 binds directly to the RBD if antibodies fail to block its interaction. Receptor-ACE2 binding domain interactions are detected and measured at 450 nm. The authors stated that this technique significantly saves time, as they obtained their results in about 4 hours compared to viral neutralization assays. Unlike molecular diagnostic techniques, serological methods can detect the presence of the virus even in samples with a lower viral load or in asymptomatic patients. As with other tests, false-negative results are expected when testing for antibodies, possibly because lower antibody levels are undetectable given the detection threshold. Hence the results depend on the safety of the people.

CRISPR technology

CRISPR, or clustered, regularly spaced, short, palindromic repeats, is a DNA sequence discovered in the genome of prokaryotes and used as a defense mechanism against bacteriophages. A CRISPR-associated enzyme (Cas) is an endonuclease that cleaves a target nucleic acid sequence under the guidance of an RNA molecule called gRNA. After its discovery, this technology was heavily invested in genome editing for therapeutic purposes. Also, CRISPR technology can easily and accurately detect the SARS-CoV-2 gene sequence. The most common endonuclease enzymes used to target SARS-CoV-2 genes include Cas9, Cas12, and Cas13 (Behera et al., 2021). One commercially available technique is SHERLOCK, which stands for High Sensitivity Enzyme Reporter Unlocking, developed by Sherlock Biosciences. This technique combines isothermal amplification of reverse polymerase chain reaction and lateral flow assay. A study identified synthetic protein S and Orf1ab fragments using Cas13 endonucleases. According to their protocol, RNA is first extracted from nasopharyngeal or oropharyngeal swabs. cDNA is synthesized. An isothermal reverse polymerase chain reaction using specific primers to amplify the S and Orf1ab genes was performed at 42°C for 25 min. Cas13 is then added to the target along with the gRNA and cleaves the amplified sequences. A reporter RNA is also added to the mixture as a lateral flow band indicator, the cutoff of this reporter indicates the presence of virus. Finally, the lateral flow strip is immersed in the solution for 2 minutes and the appearance of two test lines means that the sample is positive. This test can detect as many as 10-10 sequences per microliter. (Zhang et al., 2020) Another technique is a combination of RT-LAMP and lateral flow assay called SARS-CoV-2 DNA endonuclease targeted CRISPR trans reporter or DETECTR. It uses Cas12 enzyme to separate E and N genes. First, they extracted RNA from clinical swab samples and performed RT LAMP with specific primer sets to amplify target genes. Then Cas12 endonuclease targets and cleaves the amplified sequences with the help of gRNA. They tested two techniques to indicate the presence of virus in a sample: fluorescence reading using single-stranded DNA (ssDNA) probes and lateral flow bands using reporter molecules. The results of both detection methods were in agreement. (Broughtonet al., 2020) Table 3 below shows examples of Cas9-12-13 and their subtypes that are used to detect SARS-CoV-2. CRISPR-based technology is advantageous because it is simple. Fast, results can be obtained within 30 minutes to 1 hour. And it's cheap because it doesn't require expensive instrumentation, so it's perfect for rapid point-of-care testing.

Biosensor-based approaches

Biosensors are devices widely used in disease diagnosis by detecting nucleic acids, proteins or biomarkers in samples. Therefore, they serve as promising candidates for the detection of viruses, including SARS.CoV-2. These devices have three main components: a transmission element, a bioreceptor element and a detection system. A transducer is a device that converts biochemical reactions into a measurable output signal, and its surface is made of a conductive material. Bioreceptor elements are molecules such as antibodies, enzymes, or nucleic acids that are immobilized on the surface of the transducer, where analytes flow and bind to these elements to induce a measurable response. The analyte-bioreceptor interaction changes the electrical signal measured by a detection system. The most widely used biosensors in viral detection applications include electrochemical and optical biosensors, which are described in the following sections.

In electrochemical biosensors, chemical changes caused by analyte binding to the bioreceptor produce an electric charge that corresponds to the concentration of the analyte and is detected by the detection system (Abid et al., 2021). Some researchers are shifting their focus to biosensor systems in SARS-CoV-2 detection because they are simple and cost-effective. For example, a biosensor for the detection of S and N antigens in samples from COVID-19 patients using a sandwich hybridization method in an electrochemical biosensor, where immobilized anti-SARS-CoV-2 antibodies bind to antigens on a conductive electrode. designed. As current passed through the solution, this interaction caused changes in voltage. They found that the technique was very sensitive compared to the gold standard, and results were obtained within 2 hours. (Chaibunet al., 2021) Another electrochemical biosensor detected S antigens using the field effect transistor detection technique, which depends on the variable electric current between two electrodes, and the accumulation of the resulting electric charge is proportional to the concentration of the analyte. Anti-SARS-CoV-2 antibodies are immobilized on the graphene transducer, and the interaction between the analyte and the antibodies releases an electrical current detected by the instrument. This technique is also highly sensitive for distinguishing SARS-CoV-2 from other coronaviruses.

In optical biosensors, a beam of light hits a conjugated prism on a transducer. The detector measures the change in refractive index of the reflected light caused by the biochemical reaction. (Abid et al., 2021) Dai et al. developed a label-free surface plasmon resonance based on laser heterodyne feedback interferometry that detects SARS-CoV-2 S protein from patient samples. This sensor measures the change in refractive index in response to antigen-antibody interactions in real time, with a detection limit of 0.08 pg/mL (Dai et al., 2022). Another optical biosensor detects IgG levels in patient serum samples using the principle of photoluminescence spectroscopy. The sensor is constructed with a semiconducting polymer layer in which an RBD-engineered antigen is immobilized, and the change in the optical spectrum of the semiconducting polymer caused by binding of the antigen to the antibody requires a droplet-sized sample volume. measures. (Bassi et al., 2022) Some examples of electrochemical and optical biosensors for SARS-CoV-2 antigen or antibody detection. The speed, sensitivity, and high specificity of biosensors make them an excellent alternative for point-of-care testing, as they provide real-time viral detection. Electrochemical biosensors may be preferred over optical biosensors because they can detect lower concentrations of analyte, while lower amounts of analyte elicit smaller responses in the latter. Also, these sensors do not require bulky equipment, can be easily miniaturized, and will be wearable for self-testing in the near future after validation.

Nano-based techniques use nanoparticles (NPs) to increase the efficiency of detecting signals that arise from antigen-antibody binding. These approaches are very attractive in the fields of viral detection because NPs are stable and biocompatible in the reaction medium. Sensors using NPs as transduction elements are fast, highly sensitive and accurate, mainly because nanoparticles such as gold (Au) are excellent conductors. Nano-based approaches include combining nanoparticles with biosensors, immunoassays, and molecular-based techniques. Nanotechnology detection methods provide practical alternatives to RTqPCR for rapid and accurate virus detection. For developing countries, magnetic nanoparticles can promote the extraction of viral RNA through coprecipitation and can be used for up to 50,000 diagnostic assays (Kevadiya et al., 2021). Fluorescent semiconductor quantum dots (QDs) are one of the most commonly used nanomaterials for biological applications. QDs are a common tool for investigating S-ACE2 protein binding stimuli and exploiting them for their properties, such as small size, biocompatibility, photostability, and ease of surface interaction with biological molecules. QDs probes can also support the detection and cell-based study of other viral receptors. Also, gold nanoparticles (AuNPs) absorb electromagnetic radiation in the visible spectrum, so they have been used as a rapid colorimetric method (10 min) to detect the N gene in SARS-

CoV-2 conjugated to AuNPs with thiol-modified antisense oligonucleotides. it depends. . After the recombinant S receptor binds to the ACE2 receptor, the fluorescence is reduced by AuNPs. (Oh et al., 2005) Gold-based nanomaterials can produce neutralizing antibodies and recombinant proteins for SARS-CoV-2 or those viruses that use S-mediated cell recognition and invasion through their surface functionalization with specific aptamers. identify S (Aithal et al., 2022). Biosensor devices have been developed by adding plasmonic metal oxide nanoparticles (Ag, Au) and bio-transistor sensors and graphene to detect viral diseases. (Farzin et al., 2020; Talebian et al., 2020) Graphene biosensors are used for the detection of SARS-CoV-2 due to their sensitivity, since S antibodies can be immobilized on the surface of graphene. (Seo et al., 2020) Conjugation of AuNPs and AgNPs to antibodies - after their binding to virus antigen or its RNA - results in a detectable signal for SARS-CoV-2 detection. (Tymm et al., 2020) In recent work, a one-step optical protein S nanoplasmonic resonance sensor has been developed. This sensor requires no sample preparation and immediately detects the virus through highly specific immunoglobulins that bind to the SARS-COV-2 S protein on the nanosensor plate, ultimately resulting in plasmon resonance that can be detected visually. . (Huang et al., 2021; Yanik et al., 2010)

Another recently developed diagnostic sensor involves a dual plasmonic photothermal action based on localized surface plasmon resonance. This detection on gold nanoislands contains specific complement receptors that homogenize with SARS-CoV-2 nucleic acids. The model is excited at two separate wavelengths; The former is from a photothermal plasmonic biosensor, while the latter comes from localized surface plasmon resonance. This biosensor detects RdRp, ORF1ab and E genes and is more accurate in multi-gene sequences with a lower detection limit (0.22 Pm), which significantly reduces false positive results. (Qiu et al., 2020) ORF1ab and N genes in patient swab samples using RT-LAMP, then dipped the lateral flow assay strip into the mixture to obtain results only one hour after sample collection. They used streptavidin-NP dye-coated polymer immobilized on the conjugate pad, which resulted in rapid detection with high sensitivity and specificity. (Zhu et al., 2020) New nanomaterial-based detection systems using smart materials have been reviewed by Kevadiya et al. (2021) and Singh et al. Kevadiya et al. (2021) and Singh et al. (2022)

NPs shape the future of detection because they are small in size but offer a high surface-to-volume ratio that allows the use of smaller amounts of analyte and hence lower detection limits when used as delivery materials. offers Also, NPs offer therapeutic options; NPs combined with drugs enable targeted drug delivery specific to SARS-CoV-2. All the mentioned features of nano-based techniques make them suitable for point-of-care testing. However, clinical trials in the diagnosis of COVID-19 using these techniques are still limited.

Ideally, diagnostic methods should be accurate, scalable, rapid, and inexpensive to allow for population-based trials. The N gene was the target of choice for many researchers who used molecular-based methods to identify SARS-CoV-2 due to its high stability. (Kudo et al., 2020; Dao Bokelmann et al., 2021; Broughton et al., 2020; Chaibun et al., 2021; Dong et al., 2021; Grant et al., 2020; Lu et al., 2020 ; Zhu et al., 2020; Thi et al., 2020) Some researchers are testing the efficiency of SARS-CoV-2 detection directly from samples without RNA isolation and found a good match compared to the standard method.

Different methods such as RT-LAMP colorimetry and RT-qPCR detected the virus in positive clinical samples (NP swabs) without prior RNA extraction and did not obtain false results. (Miranda et al., 2020; Wei et al., 2021a) However, one study showed reduced sensitivity in RT-LAMP results using direct saliva and nasopharyngeal swabs, stating that RNA isolation is a critical step for effective identification. It is a virus (Taki et al., 2021). Nevertheless, bypassing RNA isolation reduces analysis time and addresses the shortage of reagents and instrumentation for rapid universal testing in resource-limited countries, in particular. (Miranda et al., 2020) As most of the tests for Covid-19 are molecular based, more focus should be directed to serological methods as they are essential for vaccine development and identification of potential plasma donors. One issue is that it takes time to develop assays during a rapidly evolving pandemic. Today, RT-qPCR is still the most widely used, but suffers from giving false negative results in samples with low viral load, ddPCR overcomes this limitation. Research is still ongoing to develop cost-effective approaches for the diagnosis of COVID-19, especially after the global economic crisis caused by the pandemic (Jackson et al., 2021). However, authorities should consider accuracy and cost to select the appropriate detection method based on the capabilities of each region. Combining gold standard diagnostic methods will certainly validate the tests to avoid false results and their associated consequences. A review of treatment for coronavirus disease 2019 (COVID-19): therapeutic repurposing and unmet clinical needs. For the early phase of the 2019 coronavirus disease (COVID-19) pandemic, drugs that inhibit severe acute respiratory syndrome coronavirus-2 (SARS-CoV-2) in vitro have negligible or more than adequate efficacy due to limited clinical evidence. The limit is estimated. Most early clinical trials have flaws in study design, small sample size, nonrandomized design, or different timing of treatment initiation. However, well-designed studies in asymptomatic or mild cases or children with COVID-19 are scarce and are sorely needed to address the clinical need. However, a trend can be observed based on current clinical evidence. Remdesivir and favipiravir may shorten recovery time.

Lopinavir (lopinavir)/ritonavir (ritonavir) does not show the efficacy of treatment in severe patients. The triple therapy of ribavirin (ribavirin), lopinavir (lopinavir) and interferon (β-1b interferon) β-1b showed initial negative viral transformation and the main effect may be related to interferon. Some studies with small sample sizes have shown that interleukin-6 inhibitors may show clinical improvement. Noncritically ill patients may benefit from convalescent plasma transfusions in small sample size studies. and The role of hydroxychloroquine or chloroquine in the treatment and prevention of COVID-19 is unclear. Traditional Chinese medicine combination therapy with antiviral agents (eg, interferon, lopinavir, or arbidol) may be effective. reduce inflammation in severe COVID-19 patients, based on observational studies in small sample sizes and expert opinion.

Most of the published studies involved severe or critically ill patients with COVID-19. Combination therapy of antiviral agents and immunomodulatory drugs is especially reasonable for those critically ill COVID-19 patients with cytokine release syndrome. Medications to reduce cytokine secretion may not be helpful in early stage patients with mild disease or in late stage patients with critical disease. Traditional Chinese medicine with antiviral effects on SARS-CoV-2 and immune modulation is widely used for COVID-19 patients in China and is worth further studies. In this review, we aim to highlight available treatment options for COVID-19 based on current clinical evidence and to encourage specific clinical trials for children and patients with mild or early-stage COVID-19 disease.

Acute respiratory syndrome coronavirus-2 (SARS-CoV-2) is a novel lineage of beta-coronavirus that is genetically closely related to the bat SARS-related coronavirus (Chakraborty et al., 2020a). Since the outbreak of acute respiratory syndrome coronavirus-2 (SARS-CoV-2) in China by the end of 2019, 32,110,656 cases have been reported worldwide, and the virus has killed 980,031 people, which is 3.05% of the infected population by September 25. constitutes 2020. To date, no effective vaccines and promising antiviral agents have been developed for SARS-CoV-2, and currently available drugs are still under investigation. Therefore, many critically ill patients are treated with off-label antiviral drugs. Many drugs in emergency use are based on laboratory evidence or expert opinion. The clinical spectrum of COVID-19 ranges from asymptomatic carrier status or mild respiratory disease to severe pneumonia (Lai et al., 2020). COVID-19 tends to severely affect elderly patients with underlying medical conditions (Lai et al., 2020). In critical patients, lymphopenia, exhausted lymphocytes, and activation of the immune system due to simultaneous cytokine release syndrome lead to severe tissue damage (Cao, 2020b). Anti-inflammatory drugs may have a therapeutic role in this stage of the disease. The publication of studies on COVID-19 has been fast-tracked. Notably, two articles on the use of hydroxychloroquine (or chloroquine) for COVID-19 in the New England Journal of Medicine and Lancet were retracted due to questionable data sources (Mehra et al. , 2020a; Mehra et al., 2020b)

Because no specific treatment is available for SARS-CoV-2, the recommended treatment is based on previous experience with SARS or Middle East Respiratory Syndrome (MERS) coronaviruses. These therapeutic molecules such as viral methyltransferase inhibitors, nitazoxanide, protease inhibitors (such as lopinavir/ritonavir), interferon, therapeutic peptides, RNA synthesis inhibitors (such as ribavirin, flavirapivir, and remdesivir), anti-inflammatory drugs, traditional Chinese medicines specifically against SARS CoV-2 are not designed (Chakraborty et al., 2020c), and some are preclinical drugs that have not yet been used in humans.

Most of the drugs currently used for COVID-19 are antiviral agents or antibodies approved against diseases other than COVID-19. The conceptual antiviral mechanisms for these drugs are summarized in Figure 1. Supporting evidence from well-designed clinical trials is limited, and there is a knowledge gap between clinical settings and valid scientific evidence. It is still too early to draw conclusions about which drugs are effective against SARSCoV-2, as most studies have been carried out on an immediate basis with a limited number of patients with severe disease. For example, several trials on convalescent plasma (CP) have limited cases, non-randomized, controlled designs and targeted patients who required extracorporeal membrane oxygenation support.

Theoretically, treatment with effective antiviral agents in the early stage of COVID-19 may yield additional benefits. Agents with anti-inflammatory properties may be useful in addition to the administration of antiviral drugs for critically ill COVID-19 patients with features of cytokine release syndrome.

Therefore, both the severity of the disease and the time of initiation of treatment affect the final clinical or virological results.

In the early period of the covid-19 outbreak, although most patients with covid-19 had moderate or severe disease, they received experimental drugs only when their clinical condition worsened. There is no clinical data on treatment in asymptomatic cases or patients with mild covid-19. Although children were believed to be less susceptible to SARS-CoV-2, critical cases of COVID-19 have been reported in children (Dong et al., 2020). Further studies are necessary to fill the knowledge gap regarding acute treatment of COVID-19 in children.

Before effective antiviral drugs were available for Covid-19, current treatment options used drugs. Therefore, in this review, we aim to highlight potential therapeutic strategies from the perspective of clinicians based on updated clinical evidence, and provide a foundation for future research into effective antiviral therapies. In the future, the development of new drugs and vaccines will depend on multidisciplinary collaboration between structural biologists, chemists, and physicians. It is expected that the knowledge gap of medicine for COVID-19 will be filled if updated information is shared among global research institutions.

Drugs

Remdesivir, an RNA polymerase inhibitor, is a monophosphate prodrug that is metabolized to an active C-adenosine nucleoside triphosphate analog and exhibits activity against RNA viruses such as Coronaviridae and Flaviviridae (Siegel et al., 2017). The triphosphate form of remdesivir is a substrate of RNA-dependent

RNA polymerase complexes in coronaviruses and blocks viral RNA synthesis. The exact mechanisms of remdesivir in inhibiting RNA polymerase are discussed in the review article by Saha et al. (2020a) It shows excellent in vitro activity against several corona viruses including SARS-CoV-2 with EC50 and EC90 values of 0.77 and 1.76 μM, respectively. Remdesivir is considered a potential treatment for covid-19 early in the outbreak. (Al-Tawfiq et al., 2020; Wang M. et al., 2020). Holshue et al. Holsho et al report the first case of COVID-19 treated with remdesivir in the United States; The patient's condition improved one day after starting remdesivir (Holshue et al., 2020). However, it is unclear whether the use of remdesivir led to this improvement. Subsequently, remdesivir was used compassionately in 53 cases, of which 68% showed improvement in oxygen support, 47% were discharged, and 13% died (Grein et al., 2020).

During February to March 2020, the first randomized, placebo-controlled trial of remdesivir in China showed no virologic advantage or clinical effect in reducing recovery time and mortality compared with the placebo group. In addition, it produced several adverse effects that led to the early termination of the trial (Wang Y. et al., 2020) Other clinical trials of remdesivir are ongoing; Preliminary data from a randomized, placebo-controlled trial show that remdesivir is effective in reducing recovery time from 15 to 11 days in hospitalized patients. On April 29, 2020, the National Institute of Allergy and Infectious Diseases in the United States announced that remdesivir was superior to placebo in reducing recovery time in hospitalized patients with advanced COVID-19 and lung involvement, based on a comparative trial of the treatment of COVID-19. National Institute of Allergy and Infectious Diseases, (2020). (Beigel et al., 2020) Currently, remdesivir is being tested as a specific treatment for COVID-19 and is approved for emergency use in people with severe symptoms in the United States. (Food and Drug Organization, 2020c)

The remdesivir dosing regimen under study is a single 200 mg loading dose followed by a daily 100 mg infusion. Remdesivir showed linear pharmacokinetics in this dose range and an intracellular half-life of more than 35 hours (Sanders et al., 2020). Dose adjustment is not recommended for patients with liver or kidney dysfunction. However, remdesivir treatment is not recommended in patients with a glomerular filtration rate of less than 30 mL/min (Sanders et al., 2020). Adverse events, including gastrointestinal and liver dysfunction (increased transaminase levels), and injection site reactions have been reported to be associated with remdesivir therapy (Green et al., 2020; Mehta et al., 2020). In a placebo-controlled study, long-term 10-day courses of remdesivir treatment did not differ significantly from 5-day courses in patients with severe COVID-19 (oxygen saturation ≤94% on ambient air) who did not require mechanical ventilation. (Goldman and colleagues). ., 2020)

Favipiravir, an RNA polymerase inhibitor, is a nucleotide purine prodrug that inhibits viral replication (Saunders et al., 2020), and it showed activity against SARSCoV-2 with a high EC50 of 61.88 μM/L (Wang M and colleagues, 2020). Different dosage regimens have been suggested based on the type of infection symptom (Sanders et al., 2020). A loading dose of 2400–3000 mg every 12 hours (two doses) has been considered for the treatment of Covid-19, followed by a maintenance dose of 1200–1800 mg every 12 hours (Mentre et al., 2015 ; Sanders et al., 2020).

Favipiravir shows a tolerable safety profile in terms of overall and serious side effects compared to other drugs used for short-term treatment (Pepperell et al., 2020). Adverse effects of favipiravir, i.e. hyperuricemia (), teratogenicity (), and QTc prolongation have not been adequately studied despite its long-term and extensive use against COVID-19 (Pepperell et al., 2020). Currently, there is limited clinical experience with favipiravir for the treatment of COVID-19 (Li J. et al., 2020; Sanders et al., 2020).

In February 2020, the use of favipiravir in the experimental treatment of COVID-19 was investigated in China. In a prospective, randomized, multicenter study, favipiravir (1600 mg every 12 hours on the first day and then 600 mg every 12 hours daily, 120 subjects) was compared with umifenovir (200 mg every 8 hours daily, 120 subjects) was compared for the treatment of moderate and severe COVID-19 infections for 10 days. (Chen et al., 2020). At day 7, a difference in clinical improvement was observed in patients with moderate infection (71.4% in the favipiravir arm and 55.9% in the umifenovir arm, p 0.019). Favipiravir significantly improved the time to resolution of fever and cough. However, there was no significant difference between patients with mild/moderate disease and severe/critical disease in subgroup analysis. Additional trials are planned in more than 40 countries (Consumer News and Business Channel, 2020).

Ribavirin, a guanosine analog that has distinct antiviral mechanisms, including both indirect (inosine monophosphate dehydrogenase inhibition and immunomodulatory effects) and direct mechanisms (interference with RNA capping, polymerase inhibition, and lethal mutagenesis). (Graci and Cameron, 2006) In vitro efficacy of ribavirin against SARS-CoV-2 virus strain , WIV04 has been reported (Wang M et al., 2020). In a single-center retrospective study conducted from January to February 2020 in Wuhan, China, a total of 134 adults with severe COVID-19 were enrolled for analysis (Tong et al., 2020). Ribavirin treatment did not shorten the time to negative viral transformation, nor did it improve the mortality rate. However, in a multicenter, prospective study conducted in Hong Kong, 127 patients were randomized to a combination group (lupinavir 400 mg and ritonavir 100 mg every 12 hours, ribavirin 400 mg every 12 hours, and Three doses of eight million international units of interferon β-1b on alternate days for 14 days) or the control group (lupinavir 400 mg and ritonavir 100 mg every 12 hours for 14 days) were placed in a ratio of 2:1. (Hung et al., 2020) The median number of days from onset of symptoms to initiation of study treatment was 5 days. There was no difference in adverse events between the two groups. The results showed that the combined group from the start of combined treatment to a negative nasopharyngeal swab (7 days; interquartile range 5-11 [IQR] days) compared to the control group (12 days; IQR 8 to 15 days; hazard ratio 4.37; 95% confidence interval [CI] 1·86 - 10·24]; p = 0·001) was significantly shorter. This study suggests that early administration of combination antiviral therapy may shorten the duration of viral shedding and improve symptoms in patients with mild to moderate covid-19 (Hung et al., 2020). However, the clinical efficacy of such a combination regimen for severe COVID-19 remains unclear. Theoretically, the adverse effects of ribavirin, such as anemia, hypomagnesemia, and bradycardia, should always be remembered (Muller et al., 2007). However, neither monotherapy with ribavirin nor concomitant use with other drugs (such as interferon or lopinavir-ritonavir) for patients with covid-19 increased the incidence of pre-existing adverse events compared with controls in previous studies (Hung et al., 2020; Tang et al., 2020). In summary, the clinical efficacy and safety of ribavirin require further clinical research.

Since interferons are important cytokines that may play a role in killing virus-infected cells (Samuel, 2001), combining interferon with other antiviral agents would be a logical strategy. Interferon β-1b appears to be a key player in combination therapy based on published data (Hung et al., 2020). Therefore, future trials with combined interferon-based regimens, including different doses, types of interferon, or concomitant medications, are warranted.

Chloroquine and hydroxychloroquine

Chloroquine has been used clinically for over 70 years. It is an approved antimalarial drug; It is also used for autoimmune diseases. Laboratory studies showed that chloroquine is very effective in controlling SARS-CoV-2 infection of host cells during entry and post-entry stages. (Wang M et al., 2020)

Chloroquine's antiviral mechanisms are multifaceted. It can prevent the uptake of nanoparticles by macrophages by inhibiting the expression of phosphatidyllinositol-binding clathrin assembly protein and subsequent clathrin-mediated endocytosis. In addition, chloroquine can prevent acidification of lysosomes, thereby preventing their fusion with endocytic vesicles (Hu et al., 2020).

A small, open-label, nonrandomized trial conducted in France included 36 patients with COVID-19 (Gautret et al., 2020). Viral load in 20 subjects treated with hydroxychloroquine sulfate 200 mg three times daily for 10 days was significantly lower than untreated subjects on day 6 after entry (70.0% vs. 12.5%, p=0.0001). Notably, six cases treated with hydroxychloroquine (500 mg on day 1, followed by 250 mg/day for the next 4 days) and azithromycin achieved 100% viral clearance on day 6. (Gautret et al., 2020). In this study, 6 patients were withdrawn from the treatment arm. The endpoint of the study was throat swab viral load on day 6 after starting treatment, which was not a clinical outcome. However, study methodology and poor reporting were among the drawbacks of the study (Ferner and Aronson, 2020). Therefore, the routine use of these drugs for COVID-19 has recently been considered harmful due to side effects such as fatal arrhythmia, drug eruption, and hepatitis. A study of 84 patients with COVID-19 who received oral hydroxychloroquine (400 mg twice daily for 5 days followed by 200 mg twice daily for 5 days) and azithromycin (500 mg daily for 5 days)) received, it was done in New York. (Chorin et al., 2020) Patients admitted with electrocardiography (ECG) were followed up for an average of 4.3 ± 1.7 days. The results showed that QTc reached from the baseline mean of 435 ± 24 ms to the maximum value of 463 ± 32 ms ($p < 0.001$). Notably, 11% of patients experienced an extremely prolonged QTc (>500 ms), which may cause arrhythmia and sudden cardiac death. Therefore, hydroxychloroquine should be used with caution, especially in patients with comorbidities and those taking QT prolonging drugs. It is necessary to evaluate QTc by ECG at the beginning and after treatment. The US Food and Drug Administration (FDA) also warns against using these drugs for COVID-19 outside of a hospital setting or in a clinical trial because of the risk of heart rhythm problems (Food and Drug Administration, 2020a).

Some patients with COVID-19 develop significant inflammation with multiorgan failure requiring intensive care, and the severity and mortality of COVID-19 are associated with elevated serum cytokine levels. Notably, high levels of proinflammatory cytokines and IL-6 were observed in severe COVID-19 patients (Giamarellos Bourboulis et al., 2020; Qin et al., 2020; Wang C. et al., 2020). Such cytokine release syndrome was initiated through the JAK-STAT or MAPK/NF-κB-IL-6 pathway. Tocilizumab (TCZ), a humanized monoclonal antibody, is able to bind membrane-bound receptors and soluble receptors for IL-6 and is a potential drug for patients with severe Covid-19 (Saha et al., 2020b). Tocilizumab (TCZ), a humanized antibody targeting the IL-6 receptor (IL-6R), for the treatment of rheumatoid arthritis, juvenile idiopathic arthritis, giant cell arthritis, and chimeric antigen receptor induced by T-cell therapy. Cytokine release syndrome has been licensed. (Rubbert-Roth et al., 2018). Sarilumab, another IL-6R inhibitor for rheumatoid arthritis, and siltuximab, a chimeric monoclonal antibody against IL-6, are indicated for multicentric Castleman disease (Boyce et al., 2018; van Rhee et al., 2018).

Several retrospective, nonrandomized clinical studies reported favorable outcomes in patients treated with TCZ. A case-control study of 20 patients with Covid-19 receiving TCZ and 25 control patients reported lower mortality and/or intensive care unit admissions in the TCZ group (25% vs 72%, $p = 0.002$) (Klopfenstein et al., 2020). TCZ was associated with a lower risk of death in a before-and-after study of 85 non-intubated patients with covid-19 who had respiratory distress [hazard ratio for death: 0.035 (0.004-0.347, $p = 0.004$)] (Capra et al. .., 2020). Another cohort study of 239 patients reported a higher than expected survival rate in critically ill patients treated with TCZ (Price et al., 2020). However, a retrospective cohort study of 65 patients (32 receiving TCZ) did not show a significant difference in 28-day mortality (15% vs. 33%, p=0.15) (Campochiaro et al., 2020). In summary, many case series showed clinical improvement, radiological resolution and reduction of inflammatory markers (Morena et al., 2020; Sciascia et al., 2020; Toniati et al., 2020; Xu et al., 2020). Doses of TCZ in reported studies ranged from 80 to 700 mg per dose, usually 4-8 mg/kg, in one or two doses. Since TCZ is an immunosuppressant, its administration is sometimes associated with increased liver enzymes, thrombocytopenia, and neutropenia (Morena et al., 2020). When TCZ was administered with methylprednisolone at a dose of 1 mg/kg/day, a significant risk of bacteremia was reported (Giacobbe et al., 2020).

Other IL-6 inhibitors, such as siltuximab and sarilumab, have been reported as salvage therapy for COVID-19. Siltuximab 11 mg/kg (one or two doses) was administered to 21 patients with Covid-19 on continuous positive airway pressure therapy or non-invasive ventilation, and 76% showed clinical improvement or stable condition (Gritty et al., 2020). Sarilumab was administered at a dose of 400 mg followed by 200 mg twice in subsequent days in eight patients, and seven of them survived to discharge (Benucci et al., 2020).

As the current evidence supporting the use of IL-6 inhibitors for the treatment of COVID-19 is weak, professional societies do not recommend its use outside of clinical studies (Alhazzani et al., 2020; Bhimraj et al., 2020). Dozens of randomized, placebo-controlled trials of IL-6 inhibitors, such as clazakizumab, tociluzmab, sarilumab, or olokizumab, are underway (ClinicalTrials.gov, 2020), and Summarized in Table 1 and updated to September 2020 research. The results of these studies are expected to fill the knowledge gap in the efficacy of IL-6 inhibitor treatment for patients with COVID-19.

Inactivating antibody administration for infectious diseases was introduced in the 1890s and was largely replaced by antimicrobial agents in the 20th century (Casadevall and Scharff, 1995). CP became a treatment option for severe viral diseases such as SARS, Middle East Respiratory Syndrome, influenza A H1N1/2009, and Ebola virus disease with variable results, as no specific treatment was available for these diseases (Cheng et al., 2005; Yeh et al., 2005; Hong et al., 2011; Mayer-Jenkins et al., 2015; van Greenzon et al., 2016).

Many doctors hope that CP injection will be effective in treating COVID-19. In addition, the FDA (US) accepted applications for expanded access and emergency single-patient use of CP (Food and Drug Administration, 2020b).

Up to 33% of patients recovered from COVID-19 produced very low titers of SARS-CoV-2 neutralizing antibodies. Therefore, neutralizing antibody testing is highly recommended for CP donors (Robbiani et al., 2020; Wu et al., 2020).

A randomized, possibly underpowered, prematurely terminated trial of 103 patients with severe or threatening covid-19 who received CP at a dose of 4 to 13 mL/kg found a significant difference in the rate of clinical improvement over 28 days did not show (9.51)% versus 43.1%, difference 8.8% [95]%, [CI: -10.4-28.0%). In subgroup analysis, only patients with life-threatening disease were more likely to improve after CP injection (hazard ratio, 2.15; 95% CI, 1.07-4.32). The 72-hour negative conversion rate of viral nucleic acid detection was higher in the CP group (87.2% vs. 37.5%, $p < 0.001$) (Li L et al., 2020).

Seven case series reported the therapeutic outcomes of CP in patients with COVID-19 with disease severity ranging from mild disease to severe respiratory failure on extracorporeal membrane oxygenation (Ahn et al., 2020; Duan et al., 2020; Pei et al. ., 2020; Salazar et al., 2020; Shen et al., 2020; Ye et al., 2020; Zhang B et al., 2020). In this series of cases, clinical improvement, radiological resolution of pneumonia and reduction of viral load were observed in most patients; However, studies with comparable groups showed less promising results. One study reported a high mortality rate in both groups (6.5 in the CP group and 15.14 in the control group), and another study showed only a slight improvement in oxygen and laboratory values (Hegerova et al., 2020; Zeng et al., 2020). The volume of CP in the above studies varied from 200 to 600 ml per time for one or two sessions. The safety of CP injection was supported by a preliminary analysis of 5,000 patients enrolled in the US FDA's expanded access program, which showed serious adverse events in 0.5% of CP recipients (Joyner et al., 2020). More than 10 randomized controlled trials have been initiated to elucidate the efficacy of CP in the treatment of COVID-19 (ClinicalTrials.gov, 2020).

At the beginning of the outbreak in China, there were no approved drugs for the treatment of Covid-19. Therefore, China's official guideline recommends traditional Chinese medicine (TCM) in combination with antiviral drugs for patients with COVID-19 (Diagnosis and Treatment Plan for Novel Coronavirus Pneumonia, 7th Provisional Edition, 2020). In China, TCM departments were set up in hospitals and some cases of COVID-19 were treated accordingly. Notably, Qingfei Paidu Decoction (QPD) is highly recommended by Chinese official guidelines for approved cases in various categories in official guidelines based on practical clinical experiences. The QPD includes 21 traditional Chinese medicines that are expected to have protective effects on various organs in addition to the lung. Of the QPD components, five are supposed to have in vitro suppressive effects on SARS virus (Yu et al., 2012; Zhang D. H. et al., 2020).

In a retrospective, single-center study conducted in Hubei Province, China between January and February 2020, 63 patients with COVID-19 treated with antiviral agents alone (n = 26) and in combination with QPD (n = 37) were taken, analyzed Xin). et al., 2020). Antiviral agents used in this study included interferon, arbidol or lopinavir. Before QPD treatment, the combined group had higher blood levels of C-reactive protein (CRP) and more pulmonary inflammation and clinical symptoms than the antiviral group. At the end of the treatment, the mortality rate, length of hospital stay and improvement of lung CT score were similar in both groups. Of note, CRP, creatine kinase, myocardial band creatine kinase, lactate dehydrogenase and blood urea nitrogen level improved only in the QPD treatment group (all $P < 0.05$). Although QPD has antiviral and anti-inflammatory potential, its precise therapeutic effect for COVID-19 remains to be elucidated, and the therapeutic efficacy requires clinical validation through well-designed randomized controlled studies.

Vaccines

In addition to antiviral agents, universal use of a COVID-19 vaccine is a promising strategy to end the current pandemic. Dozens of Covid-19 vaccines designed by different organizations are in various stages of clinical trials. Saha et al. A total of 146 Covid-19 vaccines, including live attenuated, inactivated or killed, subunit and nucleic acid-based vaccines, were involved in clinical trials (Saha et al., 2020c) and summarized the number of candidates that increase in the future. With the help of immunoinformatics, scientists can select suitable peptide sequences that are potential B or T cell epitopes to develop epitope vaccines against SARS-CoV-2 (Bhattacharya et al., 2020a; Bhattacharya et al., 2020b). Another example is a peptide vaccine against a spike glycoprotein with molecular binding on toll-like receptor 5 (TLR5), which can induce a primary innate immune response against COVID-19 (Chakraborty et al., 2020b). However, the efficacy of these candidate vaccines still needs to be confirmed.

The Covid-19 pandemic is still raging and most of the drugs currently available for Covid-19 are not specifically designed to fight SARS-CoV-2. The search for effective antiviral agents specific to SARS-CoV-2 is still ongoing. Potential drugs for COVID-19 are summarized in Table 2. Ideally, inhibiting viral replication in the early stages of COVID-19 could prevent severe complications later on. In contrast, critical cases of COVID-19 benefit from anti-inflammatory therapy combined with antiviral agents, because late-stage cytokine release syndrome is the main cause of multi-organ failure and even death. Clinical evidence shows that remdesivir can shorten the recovery time of advanced COVID-19 pneumonia. However, the clinical efficacy and safety of other agents for emergency use are debated due to limitations of study designs. IL-6 inhibitors that reduce the acute inflammation induced by cytokine release after viral infection may improve the clinical outcome of critical cases of COVID-19. Several clinical trials of IL-6 inhibitors have been conducted for severe COVID-19 patients. It is too early to draw conclusions until more evidence is available from well-designed clinical trials. Traditional Chinese herbs are worth further research. However, the precise antiviral mechanisms of traditional Chinese medicines remain elusive because regimens often contain multiple components. In addition, their therapeutic efficacy requires specific evaluations based on well-designed clinical studies. Although the supporting evidence for other antiviral agents and convalescent plasma is less than that for remdesivir, the clinical use of the aforementioned therapies may still be considered in the real world for patients with severe covid-19, in the absence of contraindications. Because of limited treatment options.

In summary, a Covid-19 vaccine is the most promising strategy to end the current epidemic in addition to antiviral agents. Designing novel antiviral agents that are specific for SARS-CoV-2 will provide more effective treatment for COVID-19 patients. The development of effective vaccines and antiviral drugs both requires multidisciplinary collaboration. Before effective vaccines and antiviral drugs are available, treatment with repurposing drugs is still mainstream. Drugs that suppress the virus may be helpful for patients in the early stages of COVID-19. Agents with anti-inflammatory properties may be useful in addition to the administration of antiviral drugs for critically ill COVID-19 patients with features of cytokine release syndrome. Traditional Chinese medicines may have advantages in immunomodulatory and viral suppression aspects when administered with other antiviral agents.

Reference:

Zhou P, Yang X-L, Wang X-G, Hu B, Zhang L, Zhang W, et al. A pneumonia outbreak associated with a new coronavirus of probable bat origin. nature. 2020;579(7798):270-3.

Li Y, Yao L, Li J, Chen L, Song Y, Cai Z, et al. Stability issues of RT?PCR testing of SARS?CoV?2 for hospitalized patients clinically diagnosed with COVID?19. Journal of medical virology. 2020;92(7):903-8.

Huang P, Liu T, Huang L, Liu H, Lei M, Xu W, et al. Use of chest CT in combination with negative RT-PCR assay for the 2019 novel coronavirus but high clinical suspicion. Radiology. 2020;295(1):22-3.

Hase R, Kurita T, Muranaka E, Sasazawa H, Mito H, Yano Y. A case of imported COVID-19 diagnosed by PCR-positive lower respiratory specimen but with PCR-negative throat swabs. Infectious Diseases. 2020;52(6):423-6.

Kucirka LM, Lauer SA, Laeyendecker O, Boon D, Lessler J. Variation in false-negative rate of reverse transcriptase polymerase chain reaction–based SARS-CoV-2 tests by time since exposure. Annals of internal medicine. 2020;173(4):262-7.

Mao X, Ma Y, Zhang A, Zhang L, Zeng L, Liu G. Disposable nucleic acid biosensors based on gold nanoparticle probes and lateral flow strip. Analytical chemistry. 2009;81(4):1660-8.

Damborsk? P, Koczula KM, Gallotta A, Katrl?k J. Lectin-based lateral flow assay: proof-of-concept. Analyst. 2016;141(23):6444-8.

Ishii J, Toyoshima M, Chikae M, Takamura Y, Miura Y. Preparation of glycopolymer-modified gold nanoparticles and a new approach for a lateral flow assay. Bulletin of the Chemical Society of Japan. 2011;84(5):466-70.

Jorgensen P, Chanthap L, Rebueno A, Tsuyuoka R, Bell D. Malaria rapid diagnostic tests in tropical climates: the need for a cool chain. American Journal of Tropical Medicine and Hygiene. 2006;74(5):750-4.

Varki A. Biological roles of glycans. Glycobiology. 2017;27(1):3-49.

Connor RJ, Kawaoka Y, Webster RG, Paulson JC. Receptor specificity in human, avian, and equine H2 and H3 influenza virus isolates. Virology. 1994;205(1):17-23.

Mar?n MJ, Rashid A, Rejzek M, Fairhurst SA, Wharton SA, Martin SR, et al. Glyconanoparticles for the plasmonic detection and discrimination between human and avian influenza virus. Organic & biomolecular chemistry. 2013;11(41):7101-7.

Qing E, Hantak M, Perlman S, Gallagher T. Distinct roles for sialoside and protein receptors in coronavirus infection. MBio. 2020;11(1):e02764-19.

Hulswit RJ, Lang Y, Bakkers MJ, Li W, Li Z, Schouten A, et al. Human coronaviruses OC43 and HKU1 bind to 9-O-acetylated sialic acids via a conserved receptor-binding site in spike protein domain A. Proceedings of the National Academy of Sciences. 2019;116(7):2681-90.

Li W, Hulswit RJ, Widjaja I, Raj VS, McBride R, Peng W, et al. Identification of sialic acid-binding function for the Middle East respiratory syndrome coronavirus spike glycoprotein. Proceedings of the National Academy of Sciences. 2017;114(40):E8508-E17.

Kwon PS, Oh H, Kwon S-J, Jin W, Zhang F, Fraser K, et al. Sulfated polysaccharides effectively inhibit SARS-CoV-2 in vitro. Cell discovery. 2020;6(1):1-4.

Lundquist JJ, Toone EJ. The cluster glycoside effect. Chemical reviews. 2002;102(2):555-78.

Kiessling LL, Gestwicki JE, Strong LE. Synthetic multivalent ligands as probes of signal transduction. Angewandte Chemie International Edition. 2006;45(15):2348-68.

Branson TR, McAllister TE, Garcia?Hartjes J, Fascione MA, Ross JF, Warriner SL, et al. A protein?based pentavalent inhibitor of the cholera toxin B?subunit. Angewandte Chemie. 2014;126(32):8463-7.

Becer CR, Gibson MI, Geng J, Ilyas R, Wallis R, Mitchell DA, et al. High-affinity glycopolymer binding to human DC-SIGN and disruption of DC-SIGN interactions with HIV envelope glycoprotein. Journal of the American Chemical Society. 2010;132(43):15130-2.

Richards S-J, Gibson MI. Optimization of the polymer coating for glycosylated gold nanoparticle biosensors to ensure stability and rapid optical readouts. ACS Macro Letters. 2014;3(10):1004-8.

Jeyaram R, Priyadarzini T, Radha CA, Shanmugam NS, Ramakrishnan C, Gromiha MM, et al. Molecular dynamics simulation studies on influenza A virus H5N1 complexed with sialic acid and fluorinated sialic acid. Journal of Biomolecular Structure and Dynamics. 2019.

Sun X-L. The role of cell surface sialic acids for SARS-CoV-2 infection. Glycobiology. 2021.

Tabari MAK, Khoshhal H, Tafazoli A, Khandan M, Bagheri A. Applying computer simulations in battling with COVID-19, using pre-analyzed molecular and chemical data to face the pandemic. Informatics in Medicine Unlocked. 2020;21:100458.

Alfassam HA, Nassar MS, Almusaynid MM, Khalifah BA, Alshahrani AS, Almughem FA, et al. Development of a Colorimetric Tool for SARS-CoV-2 and Other Respiratory Viruses Detection Using Sialic Acid Fabricated Gold Nanoparticles. Pharmaceutics. 2021;13(4):502.

Medhi R, Srinoi P, Ngo N, Tran H-V, Lee TR. Nanoparticle-based strategies to combat COVID-19. ACS Applied Nano Materials. 2020;3(9):8557-80.

Abo-Zeid Y, Ismail NS, McLean GR, Hamdy NM. A molecular docking study repurposes FDA approved iron oxide nanoparticles to treat and control COVID-19 infection. European Journal of Pharmaceutical Sciences. 2020;153:105465.

Eftekhari A, Alipour M, Chodari L, Maleki Dizaj S, Ardalan M, Samiei M, Sharifi S, Zununi Vahed S, Huseynova I, Khalilov R, Ahmadian E. A comprehensive review of detection methods for SARS-CoV-2. Microorganisms. 2021 Jan 22;9(2):232.

Broughton JP, Deng X, Yu G, Fasching CL, Servellita V, Singh J, Miao X, Streithorst JA, Granados A, Sotomayor-Gonzalez A, Zorn K. CRISPR–Cas12-based detection of SARS-CoV-2. Nature biotechnology. 2020 Jul;38(7):870-4.

Tuaillon E, Bollore K, Pisoni A, Debiesse S, Renault C, Marie S, Groc S, Niels C, Pansu N, Dupuy AM, Morquin D. Detection of SARS-CoV-2 antibodies using commercial assays and seroconversion patterns in hospitalized patients. Journal of Infection. 2020 Aug 1;81(2):e39-45.

Wernike K, Keller M, Conraths FJ, Mettenleiter TC, Groschup MH, Beer M. Pitfalls in SARS?CoV?2 PCR diagnostics. Transboundary and Emerging Diseases. 2021 Mar;68(2):253-7.

Essler JL, Kane SA, Nolan P, Akaho EH, Berna AZ, DeAngelo A, Berk RA, Kaynaroglu P, Plymouth VL, Frank ID, Weiss SR. Discrimination of SARS-CoV-2 infected patient samples by detection dogs: a proof of concept study. PLoS One. 2021 Apr 14;16(4):e0250158.

Sakr R, Ghsoub C, Rbeiz C, Lattouf V, Riachy R, Haddad C, Zoghbi M. COVID-19 detection by dogs: from physiology to field application—a review article. Postgraduate Medical Journal. 2022 Mar 1;98(1157):212-8.

Nasiri K, Dimitrova A. Comparing saliva and nasopharyngeal swab specimens in the detection of COVID-19: A systematic review and meta-analysis. Journal of Dental Sciences. 2021 Jul 1;16(3):799-805.

Landa G, Miranda-Calderon LG, Sebastian V, Irusta S, Mendoza G, Arruebo M. Selective point-of-care detection of pathogenic bacteria using sialic acid functionalized gold nanoparticles. Talanta. 2021 Nov 1;234:122644.

Publisher: Eliva Press Global Ltd

Email: info@elivapress.com

Made in United States
Orlando, FL
04 November 2026

90201145R00046